I0469555

NO ROOM FOR SHAKY HANDS

How You Can Take Your Surgical Performance to the Highest Levels

By

Dr. Hugo Van Cleynenbreugel

Copyright © 2013 Dr. Hugo Van Cleynenbreugel
All rights reserved

ISBN: 1481819739
ISBN-13: 978-1481819732

No part of this book may be reproduced in any form or by any
electronic or mechanical means including information storage
and retrieval systems, without permission in writing from the
author. The only exception is by a reviewer, who may quote short
excerpts in a published review.

The information presented herein represents the views of the
author as of the date of publication. This book is presented for
informational purposes only. Due to the rate at which conditions
change, the author reserves the right to alter and update his
opinions at any time. While every attempt has been made to
verify the information in this book, the author does not assume
any responsibility for errors, inaccuracies, or omissions.

Here's how *No Room for Shaky Hands* can help you achieve better results every time you take a patient into surgery:

• It's not a theoretical text or a set of rules or protocols. *No Room for Shaky Hands* takes a down-to-earth holistic approach that recognizes the fact that your practice is unique and your habits as a surgeon are highly individual. There are no one-size-fits-all solutions, but an approach to surgery that seeks to optimize your skills and your specialty.

• Your OR is a microcosm. This means that it has three characteristics: it's a relatively isolated and closed environment, it's got a complex system of active components, and it's focused on a measurable output. I'll show you how to define your microcosm and bring it to its highest level of performance and quality.

• The book is packed with actual situations that you've probably encountered, from disoriented patients to OR assistants who just don't seem to be up to speed. I'll show you how you can take these challenges in stride and keep the quality of your service as high as possible.

• Every surgeon experiences stress, boredom, or other emotional factors that can throw you off your stride. They can range from minor annoyances to career-killing impediments. This book will help you to recognize and deal with these issues – not by ignoring them but by helping you to focus your energy on those things at which you excel.

• Most surgeons won't admit it, but surgery is a physical activity and you need to be in top shape every time you enter the OR. I reveal secrets for how to listen to your body, keep your edge, and at the same time not drive yourself crazy with worry about your performance.

• How many mistakes can be avoided with proper planning? *No Room for Shaky Hands* will show you how to prepare for surgery, cover all the possible pitfalls, and ensure that from the moment the patient is rolled into the OR the operation will proceed like a perfectly calibrated machine.

• Let's face it – sometimes you need to correct an errant OR assistant. I'll reveal the best ways to talk to your staff and elicit positive results. You don't need to play the "blame game" to ensure accountability, and this book will show you how.

• Mistakes will happen. The goal of every surgeon is to minimize their severity and make every effort to ensure that the same mistake doesn't happen twice. I'll discuss the importance of checklists – just like commercial airline pilots have used for decades – and of reviewing procedures to eliminate the sources of mistakes.

• Surgery – indeed, any medical procedure – is a blend of art and science. It's the human hand wielding the steel blade. It's the eye following the reading on the gauges. It's the ear hearing the sounds of the OR during the operation. I discuss why it's important for every surgeon, and everyone in the OR, to approach surgery with both technical skill and an open heart (no pun intended).

• Risk is everywhere. Your OR could flood; an assistant could make a mistake; the power could go off in the middle of a four-hour operation. You can't escape risk but you can minimize it and prepare for it. And the more you can think ahead, the less stressed you'll be when you scrub up for work.

• Above all, when you're a surgeon you want to focus all of your attention and energy on helping your patients get better and live longer, healthier lives. *No Room for Shaky Hands* can help you do just that – every day, every patient, every operation.

CONTENTS

PREFACE

They say everybody has a book inside of them. I don't necessarily believe that's the case. I believe everybody has good ideas that are worth sharing. I believe everybody has his or her own truth and a personal, peculiar way of looking at the world around them; and that everybody has good insights. But the enormous amount of grit one needs to go from a good idea to a book has surprised me. I've found that to actually write a book you need a very good reason, and if possible several good reasons.

I guess for every author it's different. For me, it was clearly one thing that initiated this whole idea of writing a book, and that was to make a tiny little difference. To have the ability to affect change.

When I was writing I had no idea who would read this piece of work or who would be influenced by it. Would it sell five copies or five million? There was no way of knowing when I was slaving away behind my computer.

But in any event, I knew this book would change something. There would be a new offering on Amazon. The Google search results when typing in "operating room" and "human performance" would change. The used-disk space on my backup drive would change. The keyboard of my laptop would change by the wear and tear of my fingertips.

And most of all, I would change.

To me, writing this book has been the great escape from the routine and the rat race. Writing a book is hard, frustrating, and time consuming, but there is one thing that it's not. It's not one-on-one, whereas the rest of my work is. You see, what physicians do is mostly one-on-one. There is one doctor helping one patient with one treatment. One surgeon, one patient, one surgery. We do the one-on-one trick again and again, sometimes fifty times a day, because we have almost no leverage. It's not scalable. You can't do five operations at once. A lot of the work needs to be done by us and it's very difficult to outsource to others.

Not that there is something intrinsically wrong with one-on-one. The work I get to do as a doctor and surgeon is most rewarding. The one-on-one doctor-patient relationship is in fact the most important aspect of my work, and since I have the chance of giving people better eyesight it's the best job in the world. But to do something that's not one-on-one is also liberating. Writing a book means I can write once and reach many.

In his book *Better: A Surgeon's Notes on Performance*, Atul Gawande describes this perfectly: "Write something. I do not mean this to be an intimidating suggestion. It makes no difference whether you write five paragraphs for a blog, a paper for a professional journal, or a poem for a reading group. Just write. What you write need not achieve perfection. It need only add some small observation about your world....You should not underestimate the power of the act of writing itself. I did not write until I became a doctor. For all its complexity, medicine is more physically than intellectually taxing. Because medicine is a retail enterprise, because doctors provide their services to one person after another, it can be a grind. You can lose your larger sense of purpose. But writing lets you step back and think through a problem.

Even the angriest rant forces the writer to achieve a degree of thoughtfulness. Most of all, by offering your reflections to an audience, even a small one, you make yourself part of a larger world. Put a few thoughts on a topic in just a newsletter, and you find yourself wondering nervously: Will people notice it? What will they think? Did I say something dumb? An audience is a community. The published word is a declaration of membership in that community and also of a willingness to contribute meaningful to it. So choose your audience. Write something."

Why did I write this book? Why was I the one who decided that this message should be shared? I am someone who has spent a lot of time in the operating room (OR). I have a low complication rate. Statistics show that I am efficient and fast. However, a lot of surgeons do exactly what I do. Some do it even better! The thing of it is, most of them do it intuitively. The difference between me and other experienced surgeons seems to be the fact that for one reason or another I'm able to pinpoint what makes the difference between good and excellent human performance. I like to make surgical performance quantifiable.

To help me do this, I carry notebooks. I discovered a long time ago that trusting my memory is a naïve and stupid thing to do. No matter what your background, IQ, or education, the human memory is a sieve. So I equipped myself with a notebook, a pen, and a digital camera; and even today if I happen to leave the house without them I make sure that I process whatever I have jotted town on the napkins I bring home with me afterwards.

Indeed, the intuition of experienced surgeons can be a handicap. Some surgeons even "lose" it. At a certain moment in their career, they suddenly lose their flow, their mojo, their cool. Sometimes they lose it following an adverse or serious event. But sometimes it just evaporates, following nothing in particular.

At a certain point I decided that because of this intuition, my audience needed to be not only residents and young surgeons, but all surgeons,. If I could make things better – even a little bit – it would make all the long hours of writing worthwhile.

I believe writing makes me a better person. Every writer has woken up in the middle of the night thinking, "After all this time I spent writing this stuff, what if it's all just a pile of cow poo?" You need to stand tall. You need to get your word out there and keep your fingers crossed. You need to be confident. There is no other way than to first put in the long lonely hours and then see what happens.

INTRODUCTION

This book is about human performance. In particular, by surgeons.

Why do some surgeons perform better than others? Ever since I became intrigued by this question, my interest has grown and is still growing. The main puzzle is the question of how people function at their best in demanding situations, and to me this has been like a virus for which I have found no cure. A couple of years ago, as I delved more and more into human performance, people started to ask me to give lectures about this subject. Initially, the content that I presented in my lectures was a mixture of literature and my own experiences.

But the more I spoke to people about the prevention of medical mistakes, the more I came in contact with the most real and authentic source of information: the corridors.

It's really amazing how many people have approached me in hospital corridors to have an informal chat, just to tell their story. Times are changing. Surgeons don't want to sit on the fence any longer, being subject to whatever opinions hospital management, courts of law, or the media might have. There's a genuine need to open up the discussion about medical mistakes and how to improve human performance in operating rooms. People are willing to share their stories and I can honestly say that thanks to all of the stories I've heard and gathered, this book is based not only on the available literature and my own experiences but also on stories and experiences shared with me.

All the names in this book have been altered, but all the stories are real and are presented truthfully. I consider myself lucky that I've been able to create this book, and it's thanks to the many conversations I've had with people in the past few years.

As far as I know, surgeons are among the most action-minded people on this planet. Therefore I haven't written a theoretical work but more of a how-to book. Most of the literature that's available on the subject of human performance in operating rooms uses the "eagle eye" viewpoint. Mostly it's described from a distance: how the system works and how it can be improved. Like looking at things from the air, most literature and training programs try to capture the bigger picture. Hence, the explanation of the way people ought to fit into this bigger picture is no more than a logical corollary.

The main purpose of this book is different. Although this book also assesses the overlying bigger picture, I felt that there was a real need to talk about the "mouse eye" viewpoint. So the focus of this work is different than most other books. What I want to do is to give you, the reader, answers to these questions: What can you do? How can you make a difference? How do you fit in? How can you cope with the stress and struggle that sometimes comes with working in the operating room? In the practical way, what's your role? How about you – yes, you!

This is not a book simply and solely for surgeons. This book is for everyone who works in the operating room. I think it could be a good read for everyone working in a hospital. Hopefully it could be even of use for all fields where human performance is involved. However, while I was writing this book, I started to notice that the only way to express my thoughts accurately was to write it from my own viewpoint as a surgeon. So although

I don't necessarily consider this to be a book solely written for surgeons, I'm convinced that the fact that is clearly written by a surgeon benefits the content.

Also, this book is very incomplete. The field of human performance is so extremely complex that you could fill a whole library with books about the topic and still you wouldn't have covered every detail, every possible opinion, and every piece of research. The good news is you don't need to know every single word that has ever been written. Focus on what needs to be fixed first. If you do that you'll improve your work tremendously. You need the words that matter, the words of the people in the field, the words that cover the most important issues. What I've described here are answers to the most important things that can go wrong. I've explicitly focussed on the shortcomings that I see happen frequently or the ones that have the most devastating impact when they occur.

In any event, this book is written for "doers." For people who are not waiting for lengthy observations and theoretical explanations. For people who want to get straight down to business and need compact, concrete information. This is also the reason why this is not a six-hundred-page piece of work. My purpose has always been to bundle everything I want to tell into a book that can be read on a direct flight from Amsterdam to New York. I really hope that at the end of your journey, when its time to store your book back into your hand luggage, you think back at the flight and have the feeling of being wiser and smarter than at take off.

1. THE MICROCOSM SYSTEM

The Art and Science of Surgery

I kindly ask you to do me one small favor.

Forget the way you're used to reading literature in your field of surgery. Forget the way textbooks look. Forget how you're used to seeing medical papers. Forget about the introduction, methods, results, discussion and literature lists.

Not that there is something wrong with the way medical papers are designed. *Au contraire!* The typical design we are used to seeing in medical papers and textbooks is perfect to present to us the scientific data they're describing. However, they are not always fun to read. An even more, with typical medical literature, it's sometimes hard to use the information "tomorrow morning on the workfloor," as they say.

This is a different kind of book.

I don't ask you to believe me with blind faith, but this book will show you how you can immediately begin to decrease the chances of anything going wrong in your operating room.

Not after you have written new protocols. Not after you have discussed things in the operating room committee.

No, tomorrow morning. The only thing you have to do is to believe me when I say that different writing styles aim for different goals. The writing style of this book aims to be fun and easy to read, and to be applicable tomorrow morning. The only thing you'll have to do is to be open to the fact that the writing style is casual and friendly. You won't find the typical crammed tables, endless footnotes, and mountains of p-values. Believe me, what this book is going to teach you won't fit in this kind of format.

This book discusses human performance in the operating room. And whether we like it or not, a large part of this is the avoidance of mistakes. The fewer mistakes that are made in the operating room, the better our overall results will be and the more lives we can improve or even save.

Now, talking about medical mistakes is tricky. Besides legal and ethical concerns, nobody likes to talk about their mistakes. Most of us would rather pretend they never happen and we certainly don't like to drag them up, which is only human. And yet the best way to learn to stay out of trouble in our OR is to talk about previous mishaps. Moreover, talking about mistakes is not only useful, it also has a soothing effect. Compare it to going to the confessional, if you will. It's the confession that matters, not the priest who dispenses absolution. Sharing something that you feel you need to confess can give an enormous feeling of relief. The main difference, however, is the fact that the confessional at church is a one-way event. One person is talking and the other listening. In medicine we should try to create an atmosphere of trust, a feeling of safety, that invites people to talk freely.

And someone has to go first. Someone needs to be the first to open up.

So why not me?

The majority of my time is spent working in the operating room where, amongst other things, I perform corneal transplants. This type of operation is carried out on people whose vision has become considerably impaired, and involves replacing the cornea – in layman's terms the clear curved part in the very front of the eye – which has become cloudy. The tissue which is used to replace the diseased, cloudy part of the cornea is taken from those people who have been generous enough to donate their corneas upon their own death. Before it can be used, it first has to be processed, prepared, and checked for quality in a special kind of laboratory known as a cornea bank. As you might imagine, the requirements in terms of quality are extremely high, and if there is even the tiniest element of doubt that the tissue might not be suitable, it cannot and will not be used.

On the day before a cornea operation is due to take place, the donor replacement tissue is transported from the cornea bank to the hospital. The donor cornea is stored and delivered in a bottle containing a special liquid, and the bottle itself is packed inside a protective box so that it's cushioned from any accidental blows and stands the greatest chance of arriving at the operating room unharmed. This special box carries a great big, fluorescent sticker that says "Do Not Refrigerate" in four different languages. It's not exactly the type of sticker which could be easily missed.

On one particular morning, I arrived at the operating room to carry out two scheduled cornea transplants that were to be performed within the space of three and a half hours. Upon my arrival, the first of the two patients had already been prepared and was awaiting surgery, but the box containing the donor tissue wasn't in the cabinet where it was supposed to be, a fact which made me feel instantly uneasy. There was, however, a refrigerator in the same room as the cabinet and, sure enough, this contained the box with its large, fluorescent sticker declaring "Do Not Refrigerate." Two perfectly healthy corneas that had been processed, prepared and quality-checked in advance had been sitting in the refrigerator overnight and were now totally unusable for the purposes of transplantation.

Even though there is an extensive protocol for the delivery of donor tissue at the reception; even though every member of staff who works at the reception had been trained in these protocols and in how to accept donor tissue; despite the big, luminous sticker in four different languages and the fact that everything had gone smoothly a thousand times before, somebody had taken the box from the taxi driver, signed for the delivery and, in a brief moment of mental shortsightedness, placed the box in the refrigerator.

By the time the lost tissue and the lost time in the operating room (which was now unused for the entire morning) were taken into account, the estimated financial cost of this person's "blip" amounted to about 20,000 euros ($25,400). This, however, wasn't the worst of it, because of course the cost to those two people who didn't get their transplants was incalculable! And guess who had to deliver the bad news to the patients? That's right... me!

Have you ever found yourself in this weird situation: there are ten people in a room, and then something goes wrong and the number instantly drops to two.

"Hey," you think, "Where did everybody go?"

Now it's only you and the patient. Nobody else. Only you and the patient, and a lot of bad news to be explained.

In the wake of this incident, of course the protocols for accepting donor tissue had to be re-evaluated (yet again), and now *two* people have to verify the name, date, and details, and ensure that the tissue is properly stored. While this new system still cannot offer a cast-iron guarantee that nothing will ever go wrong in the future, it has reduced the chance of future mistakes by a factor of one hundred! Both of the patients who should have received their transplants on that day were successfully operated on shortly afterwards, but of course what happened still left a bad aftertaste for everyone concerned.

As a result of the events of that fateful day, what we learned was that even a process as simple as accepting a box and storing it in the right place will not always go as it should. More importantly though, what we discovered was that the word "Refrigerate," despite being preceded by "Do Not," was what had actually caused the problem, as this was the word that had stuck in the individual's mind. Not only was this a very surprising discovery, but it was also frightening to realize just how easy it is to develop a blind spot for something despite big warning signs and safety labels. How could something so simple go wrong, and right under our very noses?

So, how on earth can we get a grip on human performance and stay out of trouble in our operating room? The avoidance of surgical mistakes is a difficult subject to get your head around because it's complex. The days that surgery was a simple thing are long gone, if those days ever existed. In *Blood and Guts: A History of Surgery*, Richard Hollingham describes beautifully how in the beginning of the nineteenth century, surgery was done with only a couple of sponges, a knife, a saw, and some threaded needles, with a smoky coal fire burning in the corner of the operating room.

Often, the operating theatre would be positioned at the centre of the hospital. It was separated from the public areas by thick walls and it was not accessible to the general public. This arrangement had two significant advantages: it helped shield passers-by from the screams of patients being in surgery, which would only upset the other patients and visitors in the hospital. Second, even in the early days of surgery, it had become obvious that it was easier for surgeons to focus on the task at hand when they had their own room, separated from the rest of the hospital (that's right, a microcosm indeed, thank you for noticing).

If possible, the operating room was located next to the morgue. Its proximity to the mortuary meant that after their surgery, surgeons could easily go there to study anatomy and get some post-mortem practice.

Not infrequently they would do surgery and post-mortem training on the same unlucky patient.

1. THE MICROCOSM SYSTEM

And since it was often unclear what the actual outcome of the surgery would be, there was little discussion about medical mistakes. You cannot talk about an undesired end result if you don't know what the end result should be exactly.

Anyway, it's clear that times are different now. Surgery has become increasingly more complex and yes, when we operate we definitely have a clear vision of the desired end result. So discussions about medical mistakes are more alive than ever, and great effort is being spent upon the prevention of mistakes.

But the prevention of surgical mistakes is just half the story. Look, a mistake is always something someone has either done or failed to do. There is always someone who is the culprit, who should have done things differently. Someone has messed up. And to prevent mistakes we can learn from the past. If we can make sure people won't do in the future what this someone has done in the past, we will be okay in our operating room, right? Well, of course.

Unfortunately this is not the whole story.

First, mistakes can only be made if there's no safety net to prevent them. Nobody drives to the hospital in the morning to do a bad job. We're all doing the very best we can. Let's say Jim has mistakenly injected the wrong dose of antibiotics intravenously. That's what we call a mistake, and Jim should have done things differently. Quite obvious, isn't it? But wait a minute. If Jim had acted the exact same way but there had been a safety procedure to check the dose of the antibiotic before he injected it, wouldn't that be a solution also?

7

There are always two sides to the story. If we focus on the actual mistakes only, we create the false and dangerous illusion of control. Dealing with the initial mistake is easy because it's tangible. One can easily pinpoint what went wrong, when it went wrong, and who was holding the instrument that caused the disaster.

Looking at the underlying safety mechanisms that should be in place is much more difficult, but much more valuable.

Second, learning from mistakes is overrated. You can study mistakes. You can unravel them. You can dwell upon. You can discuss them until you turn blue in the face. That's all very valuable. Mistakes that happened in the past are important lessons for the future. But seriously, what do you really learn from mistakes? You learn what not to do again. By knowing what *not* to do again, you won't necessarily know what you *should* be doing instead!

The study of failure and mistakes is not a one-way ticket to a mistake-free operating room. It's part of the solution but it's definitely not the whole story. While the improvement of the quality of the work that's being done in the operating room depends in part on the study and prevention and mistakes, not doing what's wrong is *not* the same as doing what's right.

Third, the moment you label someone as the culprit you're dooming your whole organisation to a culture of name, blame, and shame. And that is a bad place to be. Sure, in case of an error, someone should have paid more attention, someone broke the rules, someone should have spent more time in the surgical skills lab. But to put someone in the pillory is a bad idea, because other people will wonder how they can make sure they won't be put in the pillory like that when they make a mistake.

Errors can occur everywhere and anywhere. Sooner or later, everybody will be in a situation where the chances of messing up are high, and people know that. So the more you name the wrongdoer and blame him for it, the more you will encourage people to avoid responsibility. Nobody likes to stick one's neck out if making mistakes means being punished in public. And in operating rooms, where the difference between life and death can be determined by a quick and resolute clamping of the aorta, we need people who are willing to stick their neck out if necessary.

Fourth, you need to honestly ask yourself the question whether you want to see the people in your organization taking aspirins or vitamins.

I'll explain. The prevention of mistakes is the aspirin. It's solving problems. Making sure bad things don't happen. When you instruct people how they can prevent mistakes you bring them from minus one to zero. You bring them from a bad situation where problems occur (-1) to an okay situation where everything is all right (0). That's a very important thing to do, and it's definitely the first step. However, it's also a narrow-minded approach because it's only the first step and nothing more. Almost every single human being whom I have ever met in an operating room wanted to do much more than doing a job that's okay. People want to feel empowered. People want to be challenged, to be part of a greater stimulating entity. People want to be inspired by their team, and they want to be able to do something in return and to contribute. To me, empowerment means releasing the skills, motivation, and experience that's already in people. It's the creation of the right circumstances for people to thrive, to excel, to put their knowledge and talents to good use, both individually and as a team.

Empowerment is the vitamins. And we need vitamins too. Now "empowerment" is quite often used only as a nice sounding buzzword. Why? Because creating the right circumstances for empowerment is difficult. Here's the rub: one of the key factors of empowerment is the fact that people are given some degree of autonomy and the freedom to think for themselves. It means balancing between rules and freedom, between following guidelines and thinking for yourself. And in an operating room where so many rules are set in stone, this can be a very difficult balancing act. Luckily, difficult doesn't mean impossible, and it's worth the effort. When you create an atmosphere of empowerment, you bring people from zero to plus one, and this is exactly what makes the difference between an organisation that is merely "good" and one that is "excellent."

So if you want to aim for not just a good functioning operating room but one that's a pleasure to work in, you'll need a two-tier approach to things. You want both the aspirins and the vitamins. And that's what we will look at in this book. Of course those two are intimately connected, and for some of the topics we'll be discussing it won't be clear if the solution comes out of the aspirin or the vitamin box. My point is this: In any OR there is much more going on than avoiding things going wrong. We want things to right. So let's go.

Your Microcosm

Let's talk about soccer for just a minute. The date was July 11th, 2010. I was watching the FIFA World Cup final. Spain against the Netherlands. The Netherlands had several chances to score, most notably in the sixtieth minute when Arjen Robben was launched by Wesley Sneijder putting him one-on-one with Spain's goalkeeper Iker Casillas, but Casillas pushed the shot wide with an outstretched leg. Meanwhile, for Spain, Sergio Ramos missed a free header from a corner kick when he was unmarked. Four minutes before the end, a penalty shootout seemed inevitable. However, just before the end of the game, Navas sprinted into opposing territory and began a series of passes that led to Iniesta finally breaking the deadlock, scoring a half-volleyed shot after receiving a pass from Cesc Fàbregas.

Now in that split second before the winning goal, when Iniesta fixed his eyes on the ball, in the replay I noticed this certain look in his eyes. His eyes showed complete concentration but also something that we can best describe as a kind of disconnectedness. Although the whole world was watching, his world seemed to stop at the chalk lines. Could you call him on his cell phone? Could you get his attention in any way? No. His little world, the soccer field was completely separated from the outer world.

And then it hit me.

A microcosm is:

A system isolated from the outside world in which events, patterns, teamwork and activities are controlled as much as possible in order to create a certain goal or output.

Whether it's sports or surgery, or even music or acting, there is one pattern, one common denominator which runs like a red wire through all the fields where human performance is involved. To achieve maximum human performance, we create a closed little world with only one purpose, and that purpose is to let people do what they do to the best of their abilities. Whether it's a soccer pitch, cockpit, operating room, or a stage, the more we can close off the system from the outside world, the more control we have of what's happening within that system.

Furthermore, the more influence we have on what's happening within the system the more we can influence the end result. If people need to function optimally, both physical and mentally, we need to make sure that they have their own closed world.

What needs to be created is something we can best describe as a microcosm.

It's a closed off place on this planet where human performance can prosper to its best. A place where people get the best out of themselves and work together as a team.

Looking at things from this point of view, there's not such a difference between the soccer pitch of Iniesta or my operating room. However, our monthly wages are pretty different.

The general overlapping characteristics for all of these different microcosms are as follows:

Isolation. The microcosms are isolated from the outside world as much as possible. External influences can make the system unstable and negatively influence its functioning. And besides, the more compact and isolated a system is, the better it can be monitored.

1. THE MICROCOSM SYSTEM

Complex teamwork. Within the microcosm you will see that there is a complex system of active components. In the case of the OR, these components are the people, instruments, and computers, all working at the highest possible level. The microcosm includes everything from the ten-cent disposable latex glove to the multimillion-dollar diagnostic machine, and from the janitor who cleans the OR to the highly paid surgeon who directs a team. To achieve success it's necessary that all these elements work together the best they can. Training of people, improving coherence and collaboration, creating protocols – they're all designed to enable better process performance.

Output. The focus of the system lies with the output. Every microcosm has a goal and a reason for its existence. Without the output, nobody would bother organizing the microcosm in the first place. This focus on output can give a person the feeling that he or she is only a small part of the system. Everything is designed to optimize the output. How people feel personally – whether they're happy and healthy or not – plays a minor role. I know a pilot who once told me that even though she loved her job very much, she had a problem with feeling so replaceable. "If I'm not there, the plane will leave anyway. If I call in sick, replacement is arranged within thirty minutes. That does make me wonder sometimes how important I am in the whole system."

On the other hand, the fact that there is focus on output gives elements within the microcosm a very strong sense of solidarity. People feel connected by a common goal. And when people are pulling together, fantastic things can happen. Nothing is more satisfying than people working in close harmony.

Control. The key to success is having maximal control over what's happening within the system. I don't think you can teach surgeons much about control. More or less everything we do has the purpose of improving control over our operations (and with that, the result of them). We are absolute control freaks. No, we're control *addicts*. And that's also where the risk is. We take this urge to control with us when we leave our microcosm. We may physically leave the hospital behind when we go home in the evening, but I know enough surgeons who frantically try to keep the same level of control over supper, the groceries, the kid's homework, the time to depart for their tennis lessons, the board of the sailing club – you name it! I know because I'm one of them.

Satisfaction. On a personal level, working inside a microcosm is something that gives people satisfaction. At the moment that the task at hand poses challenges and people have to try their best, they can enter a state of timelessness where they feel completely absorbed by the task. This phenomenon, known as "flow," is one of the key factors to personal happiness.

Emotions. The stakes are high. Most microcosms harbor an activity with little room for error. Sometimes there is plenty of money involved. Sometimes – like in the operating room – we're dealing with patients and we cannot stand the idea of not providing the best possible care to everyone. That's the reason that every microcosm has a huge emotional component. You can see much joy from people if everything goes well but so much disappointment when things go wrong.

So yes, a microcosm can be a sports field, a cockpit, a music stage, an acting stage, a podium for public speaking, a laboratory, a submarine. Find optimized human performance and you will find a microcosm supporting and protecting this performance.

And for you? Your microcosm is the operating room.

And the output of the microcosm? The output is a healed patient, or at least a patient who is doing better than before the operation. American surgeon Logan Clendening is quoted as saying, "Surgery does the ideal thing: it separates the patient from his disease," and in a way this is true. As surgery typically removes all or part of a sick organ and sometimes replaces it with something else, if all goes well the result of the system is a healthy patient, or one who can at least live a better life. In the case of my patients, of course, the end result is that they can enjoy better eyesight. I like Clendening's viewpoint very much because it demonstrates the relationship between the microcosm and the output. Your microcosm is the place where the patient gets separated from its disease.

The moment I thought of the concept of the microcosm, something strange happened. Puzzle pieces seemed to come together. It's such a useful tool to me to understand performance. Despite the fact that I've always been an efficient surgeon, I have to admit that part of my work fell into the "trial and error" category before I fully understood the concept of microcosms. Now I understand my own functioning, and that of others, a lot better. But why would we start looking for the red wire in all of the different fields of human performance? Why aren't we only looking at the operating rooms, as this is what the subject of this book is about? Even though there are a lot of similarities between the different microcosms, is it really worth looking at the overlapping patterns?

The answer is yes! Because we can learn a lot from each other. Because we can pick up knowledge from different fields, we have the opportunity to learn, to expand, and to grow. We just shouldn't make the mistake in trying to re-invent the wheel all by ourselves. Fortunately for us there is such think as interchangeability, and the transfer of knowledge from one professional field to another.

Compared to, let's say, the aviation industry, the medical field is still wearing its children's shoes when it comes to the design of check lists and optimization of teamwork and safety. Nowadays, the use of safety check lists is taking hold in a growing number of hospitals around the world. However I can assure you that fifteen years ago, things were different. As far as I know, The Rotterdam Eye Hospital was one of the first hospitals worldwide that sent people to the aviation industry to see how to improve the security in the operating room. In an analogy with the cockpit check list, which is used by every pilot prior to take off, a new time out procedure was developed, in which for every surgery, the name, date of birth, the procedure, and the eye that needed surgery were checked. The medical staff was involved from the very beginning of this procedure, but also I do have to say that management of the hospital really played a pioneering role, not only by spending a lot of time and energy improving patient security, but also by introducing professional trainers from the aviation industry within the hospital, which at that given time was a revolutionary idea.

It's no coincidence that in the beginning of this chapter I referred to professional sports. In the area of personal performance, the functionality of people is deeply embedded within sports. Sport psychology is a science that has seen a enormous boost in the last thirty years One of the most important goals of sport psychology is to make sure that athletes need to enter a determined mental stage which is called "the zone." When athletes are in the zone, they're in an optimal phase in which they are able to perform at their best.

A former sprinter, Mark Richardson, talks about the zone like this: "It's a very strange feeling. It's as if time slows down and you see everything so clearly. You just know that everything about your technique is spot on. It just feels so effortless. It's almost as if you're floating across the track. Every muscle, every fiber, every sinew is working in complete harmony and the end product is that you run fantastically well." Sounds a lot like the way we would love to do our surgery, doesn't it?

The Three Levels of Performance

A couple of years ago I was asked to reside in an OR committee. The government had decided that every hospital needed to have a committee with a specific focus on adjusting and amending different processes in the OR. However, clear guidelines as to how the amendments needed to happen were not considered by the government. So, there we were at our first meeting in the coffee room of the OR with our cups of instant coffee. Soon it became very clear that in order to improve the logistics and processes in the OR, you first need to create a map. When you don't know where you are, you will not be able to map where you are in order to improve the situation, and you'll be stuck at the same place, as you cannot plan on getting any further then you already are.

Let's go back to the idea of the microcosm. If you want to influence the output of your microcosm, you'll need to influence what's happening within your microcosm. And to do that, first you need to know how it works. How it's organized. Over the years, different modules of human performance in highly demanding environments have been described. The problem with most of the modules is that they come up with impressive diagrams comprised of lots of key words connected by arrows and lines. To me, the largest part of these diagrams look more like a plate of spaghetti than something I can use in daily practice.

So I needed to design my own model.

Within the microcosm, there are three levels of performance: the personal level, the interpersonal level, and the organizational level. Every aspect of the different mechanisms and forces that we see in our daily practice contributes to the individual, the team, or the whole organization.

Of course these levels do not operate independently of each other. They are intimately connected and they influence each other continually. However, separating these three layers enables us to look at things from the human perspective. It shows where people fit in. Where we fit in. Instead of making people one of the many different kinds of cogs found in some models, the model I am proposing here comes from a different viewpoint. It first separates people as individuals, then as a team, and after all of that it deals with the rest (organization).

Let's look at the three different levels.

The personal level

The personal level is about how everyone is doing as an individual and how each person is functioning as an isolated "component" within the system. This is the level at which each person functions on their own. It's the layer of performance where you, as an individual, are responsible for your own actions. It's where we ourselves can make the biggest difference every second of the day. We can deliberately choose to take our responsibility and have a genuine look at what we can to contribute to the positive outcome of our work. Personal performance starts with responsibility for our own decisions, our own thoughts and assumptions, and our own functioning.

I once had a new resident in my OR. He was with me for one full day every week. After some time I thought the right time had come to let him take his first steps into surgery. I asked him to take his place behind the operating microscope. Sure enough, he had no idea whatsoever how the microscope worked. He didn't even realize that the microscope was remote-controlled by a foot pedal. I said, "Well, I would have thought that by now you would have taken the time to fiddle around with the microscope just to be prepared for the first time we would give you the opportunity to use it."

He looked me in the eyes and said with a straight face, "No. That's not my responsibility. I'm in training, so I assume that you are going to teach me everything. And that includes the microscope."

Wrong. The moment you enter an OR you have a responsibility to be prepared to do your job. Everybody – including people in training – has a certain level of functioning that is required. If you are not willing to contribute as a person, to play your role as well as you can, you have no business in the OR.

By the way, a little side note would be appropriate here. I don't want to sound pedantic, but if you're a resident, listen carefully. The most important thing you can ever do to be trained better than your peers is to go to the OR fully prepared. Become the best customer of the skills lab. Practice every single aspect of the surgery. Ask the head of the OR if it's okay to stay after the OR has finished and practice with every piece of equipment you can lay your hands on. Practice assembling scopes until you can do it blindfolded, figure out how pedals and machinery work until you know the effect of every single knob. Study to know every clamp and pair of tweezers by name. Your supervisors will notice and they definitely will more eager to teach you! For surgeons, training a resident can be hard, but working with residents who have done their homework is not. It's fulfilling.

The personal level is about you. It's about how you work. This means two things. The first is the quality of your work. How well do you do your job? Are you experienced enough and motivated enough? Do you have enough theoretical background? Do you possess the right skills, talents, and techniques to do the surgeries that are on your operating list?

The second is how you feel while you're slaving away on the shop floor. It's how you cope with the stress and the demands. How you can stay close to yourself without spending all of your energy in the first two hours of the day. How you can find the right balance between feeling relaxed yet being "on edge" enough to pay attention to every detail. It's in these questions that you can find peace of mind. There are enough surgeons who do their job very well but forget to think about themselves. Trying to pretend that you're supernatural will backfire on you in the long run.

It's a good idea to have an honest look inside once in a while and ask yourself "How am I coping?" There's a widespread mis-understanding that this represents a kind of weakness. It isn't. Taking care of yourself is a very good idea. Look, on a world-wide scale, there aren't that many surgeons around. It's a long and hard journey to eventually get to be called "surgeon." Not many people are willing to undertake this journey. By no means I want to call the people that are working in the OR different than others, but since it's only fair to look at our patients' health as something that is extremely valuable, let's look at you as the goose that lays the golden eggs. Just for a moment! Bear with me. If you are contributing – in whatever way – to people getting better, you are the goose that lays the golden eggs. Every successful surgery is valuable. It's a golden egg. And if the goose doesn't feel right? If the goose can't cope with the way the eggs need to be laid? No more eggs after a couple of years, right? Now in the telling of the goose that lays the golden eggs it's the cottager who was supposed to take good care of the goose. I propose something different. Let the goose take good care of herself. You owe it to your patients to perform well on a personal level, but you equally owe it to yourself.

The interpersonal level

The interpersonal level is about how people work together as a cohesive unit and an efficient team. Needless to say teamwork is important in the OR. The power of an effective team is in direct proportion to the accuracy of the work being done, the flow and speed, and patient safety. Committed teams can decrease operation time while improving their results. The complex, multi-dimensional and multi-disciplined nature of the OR requires a team approach. We can only treat our patients by combining the knowledge and expertise of all the individuals in the OR. A team that works as a well-oiled machine can produce results far greater than the sum of all individual efforts. The list of conditions that need to be met in order to build a solid team is long.

Trust, loyalty, openness, communication, constructive criticism, respect, and even shared coffee breaks. It's a tall order.

To me, the most important factor in building the right team spirit is the delicate balance between leadership and involvement. On the one hand, an OR needs leadership. Strong leadership. As a captain on a ship, one person needs to set out the course and have a clear vision of where the team is going. On the other hand, if this one person is followed blindly by the rest without hesitation, any mishap made by this one person will send the whole team down the drain. Further, it's impossible to create an atmosphere where people are willing to invest all of their energy if those people don't feel inspired and involved. A group consisting of one leader and a bunch of followers is a recipe for problems. People like to be kept informed and involved in whatever is going on. Only if their input is solicited will they feel part of something bigger.

The organizational level

The organizational level describes how the system functions as a whole, not just in relation to its human components but also including all technical aspects and all aspects related to time and location. It's simply everything that's above the personal level and the interpersonal level. It's everything you are left with when you don't take people in to account: medical devices, disposables, drugs, protocols, the time schedule, the operating room itself. It's the department of mechanics and logistics. It has a physical component (the place you work, the instruments and equipment you work with) but also a less tangible component (agreements, instructions, protocols, schedules).

In my eleven years of schooling, I have been exceptionally well educated in the technical aspects of surgery. After my initial years of acquiring theoretical knowledge, I had good teachers who taught me everything about the operations. When I started working as a surgeon I entered a well functioning system where people were working hard each day to further improve processes and quality.

However, nobody had taught me how to deal with the sleepless nights preceding a difficult operation. How I hated the sleepless nights! Nobody had taught me how to stay calm in stressful situations. Of course, as I did more surgery, I figured out on my own how to manage the stress, the doubts, and the shaky hands. But I would have welcomed a small handbook on how to deal with my own insecurities.

Organizations spend a lot of effort on the upper two layers. There's a lot of energy put into the organization on the big picture, the logistics of the processes, and the organizational level. Also, over the last few years I've seen a growing interest in the interpersonal level, the teamwork. Crew resource management, which is the training and improvement of the collaboration of people who belong to the same team, has become very important in aviation and is entering the field of medicine as well. The growing interest in optimizing the organizational and the interpersonal level in operating rooms is a very good thing.

I am convinced, though, that not enough attention is paid to how people are doing on a personal level.

This unbalance towards the organizational level and the interpersonal level is also reflected in the literature. Do a quick online search and have a look at the available books on human performance. There are good books around but most books only try to capture the big picture. A good deal of the work that has been written has a significant academic slant to it. And literature doesn't help me very much if it is written like this:

"The identification of operational requirements and the assessment of training needs and coordination demands are critical components in crew resource management. Therefore the assessment of crew preventable errors together with the optimization of risk management can be considered as instructional strategies designed to demonstrate an integrated methodology for improved human competence."

Or am I the only one not capable of translating this to my case of cataract surgery at eight o'clock tomorrow morning? So yes, this book has a significant slant towards the personal level. This is what I've been missing, not only in training and teaching but also in the available literature. In the overview you'll see that all three levels of performance are addressed. But in contrast to the approach of managers and directors, we won't start with the organization. We won't let the organizational level seep through the interpersonal level towards the personal level. We'll start from the personal level – from the bottom up if you will.

You don't need to write extensive reports or go to dozens of management courses to avoid mistakes and improve performance in your OR. You can start improving all three layers of performance right now. First get your own personal performance up to speed, then work on your team, and after that improve organization. You will be amazed what you can accomplish if you take a little step every day. Most people overestimate what they can do in a year but underestimate the gigantic power of small daily steps.

The only thing you need to do is to start today.

Start now.

Humans Are the Weakest Link

Watch out for people. The best way to avoid complications and mistakes in the OR is to watch out for people.

Of course we need people in the operating room, and not only to give the proverbial pat on the back to patients. We need people to hold the scalpel and to make the incision. To decide whether an appendicitis can be operated laparoscopically. To judge if there is enough supporting literature to justify the giving of antibiotics preoperative. All technical machinery – even the surrealistic Leonardo da Vinci operating robot – is an elongation of human thought, feeling and acting.

So my advice is not to "avoid all humans." (However, it's an appealing thought that under such circumstances there will be no more mindless discussions about what music will be played in the OR.) My advice is something different: watch out for humans. Be aware when you see people entering the OR. Watch out, because whether you like it or not, people and mistakes come together. If you want to stay out of trouble in the OR, watch out for humans.

There is nothing as predictable as the fact that people make mistakes. It's actually a matter of waiting. However, this does not mean that we have to accept it. We have to do the utmost to avoid errors. On one side a bit of sense of reality is not bad: no approach will make us completely goof-free. However we owe it to our patients to try to be as goof-free as possible!

In his book *Why We Make Mistakes*, Joseph T. Hallinan writes, "We all know the cliché, 'To err is human.'" And this is true enough. When something goes wrong, the cause is overwhelmingly attributed to human error: airplane crashes (70 percent), car wrecks (90 percent), workplace accidents (also 90 percent). You name it, and humans are usually to blame. And once a human is blamed, the inquiry usually stops there. But it shouldn't – at least not if we want to eliminate the error. In many cases, our mistakes are not our fault, or at least not entirely. For awe are all afflicted with certain systemic biases in the way we see, remember, and perceive the world around us, and these biases make us prone to commit certain kinds of errors.

Indeed, people are prone to make mistakes. And that's despite our good intentions. After all, I believe that everyone who sets foot in the operating room has the best intentions. In the end don't we all want one thing? We want to heal people. We can't solve all medical problems, but we at least want that every patient who leaves our OR is better off then when he or she entered. I believe that we act to the best of our abilities. Unfortunately that's not always enough. It sometimes looks like the tools that we work with – our body and brain – are programmed to mess up once in a while. We are prewired, without realizing it.

The list of built-in human foibles is long. Not all of them apply to every person, but I'm sure that among these you'll see a few that are familiar:

- We like to stick to our assumptions. (I can't be wrong.)
- We get too emotional. (Screw this hospital – I'm out of here.)
- We get our brains paralyzed by adrenalin. (What was I thinking when I grabbed that thorax needle?)

- We aren't good in handling criticism. (You better first have a good look at your own postops.)
- We get stuck in analysis-paralysis. (Let's go over this once again.)
- We can be tired, too high on caffeine or too low on sugar. (Wow, I feel weird.)
- We don't always get our priorities straight. (Whatever happens, we need to finish at five o'clock because I have tickets for the game.)
- We miscommunicate and still say, "But I told you so." (Indeed, I told you so.)
- We are too optimistic about our own skills. (I've never done it but it can't be that difficult.)
- We interpret everything we see and hear our own way. (The family didn't seem to be too upset.)
- We are too pessimistic about other people's skills. (Why do I always have to do everything myself? We take the short-cuts, even if there aren't any. (There should be a faster way – I have too many other things to do today.)
- We are bad at predicting the future. (We got away with it last week, so we'll probably be fine today also.)

Simultaneously, most surgeons will consider themselves to be nicely above average. Research shows that if medical errors are reported by surgeons themselves, the numbers are much lower than the numbers that are found in the literature. The same holds true for the missing of early signs of cancer on screening RX exams. The detection of prohibited objects by baggage screeners at the airport? Same results. We are just overly optimistic about ourselves. We clearly all know what the meaning of the word "average" is, but hey, half of the surgeons are above average and it's obvious that we're among them, aren't we?

There's no doubt that people make mistakes, it's ingrained in who we are. There are just too many neurological and physical shortcomings, loopholes, and pitfalls in our system.

That's one thing. Unfortunately, we don't fully recognize this in ourselves. That's a second, even more frightening, issue. We can see possible the human shortcomings when people are doing complex tasks like microsurgical skin grafts or flying a Boeing 747, but imagining others making mistakes is much easier than envisioning ourselves messing up. The reason for this is the fact that to do surgery, you need a certain mindset. You need to be convinced that you are the best – or at the least very, very good – at what you do. If not, you would be ethically obliged to send your patients to another surgeon! They say desperate diseases require desperate remedies, meaning that surgery needs to be done with confidence and determination.

And it's that unflagging self-confidence that can carry us too far.

Looking in the mirror and realizing that you have great potential for both success and failure is a humble thing to do. It's also an honest thing to do. It has nothing to do with weakness or self-doubt. It has to do with alertness. Being aware that mistakes are lurking, not only for your peers but also for you. That realization alone will make you a better surgeon.

The Ideal Low-Risk Scenario

So if humans are the weakest link, wouldn't it be great to have a human-free operating room? Wouldn't that save us a lot of trouble?

Picture this scenario. John is a seventy-six-year-old man with a solid gray bush of hair, and always has a smile on his face. On Tuesday morning he walks into a big multidisciplinary hospital. Today is the day it's all happening. He's having surgery on his left knee. All those years of running marathons have now taken their toll. John is getting a knee prosthesis, which will allow him to walk again without any pain.

John is walking through to the big reception hall where he can see the first sunlight glancing through the windows. He places his passport into a tall machine and is kindly requested to look into the white light. His eye is being scanned. The identity of his eye matches his passport and he is asked to place his hand in the machine. A light blue wristband is being placed around his wrist. The chip which is integrated is unique and recognized everywhere in the hospital. The machine is kindly telling him in a robot voice he needs to present himself to Section 12B.

Once he arrives the same kind of apparatus awaits him. Once again his iris is scanned, but this time not only his identity is checked with his passport but also with his wristband. From this moment everything is automated. The preparation for the surgery is executed by robots and machines. When John finally arrives in the operating room there is no human in sight. Robots and beeping machines are rolling from and forth.

A feminine – but still robotic – voice requests John to slowly count to ten as narcosis is induced.

Two hours later John awakens in recovery. The whole operation had been performed automatically by robots.

While John thinks about how wondrous it is that the placement of a knee prosthesis can be completely be executed without the involvement of one single human being, a sense of loneliness overcomes him. He hopes that his daughter and wife are waiting for him in the reception area.

In that moment a screen turns on in front of his bed with a message. Good news. The operation has been performed without complications.

As a surgeon it's very easy to list many reasons why this scenario would never work. Here are some reasons why.

• Despite the ever progressing evolution of technology it's impossible that technology would ever be able to take over this type of medical treatment. Behind every robot and machine there is still a human who has to make crucial decisions. Technology is, and stays, a sophisticated elongation of human thinking. Yes, technology is improving at an ever increasing speed, and we see how this pays off in our daily practice.

But new technology is doesn't necessarily means a lower risk of errors. It usually makes certain aspects of the surgery safer while introducing new opportunities for failure. New technology doesn't remove the potential for mistakes. Quite often it only relocates it.

• Surgery is not simply a succession of standard technical actions. Even in "standard treatments" there is a component of creativity, gut feeling, and human experience. A surgeon once told me "sometimes I have the feeling that somewhere inside me there is a built-in alarm system that can detect problems that we can't effectively perceive. It's hard to explain. Sometimes I'm very busy doing my surgery and suddenly there is something that makes me pause for a second. I ask the anaesthetist if everything is okay with the patient. I ask the nurse if everything is under control. I realise that this question seems to come out of nowhere and I always try to avoid upsetting people so I ask them with a smile. But I am very serious. Several times in the past it turned out that there *was* something wrong. A breathing tube that was not placed completely in the right way. A drip that was not performing well. It has even gotten so far that when I pause for a second and I straighten my back nowadays, the anaesthetist double checks the vital signs of the patient."

• Most systems, however ingenious they might be, are not capable of running completely independently. All systems have a certain amount of instability. If you allow technical systems to run autonomously then you know for sure that at a certain point they will deviate from the goal. Just like a car when you let go of the steering wheel on a straight highway. The question is not whether you're going to end up in the ditch. You know that for sure. The question is how long it's going to take, and that depends on how well the car is aligned. So the question is not whether the system is going to deviate; the question is how long it's going to take if you let it run autonomously.

The answer is simple – it depends on the technical ingenuity with which the system has been built. Just like the car on the straight highway that needs a small correction every mile, it is humans who will adjust and track the system. And only people can correct every complex technical process where needed. Only people can bring everything together like a patchwork, overseeing the bigger picture and adjusting where needed.

• Especially when complications arise, human creativity can make the difference between a good outcome and a catastrophe. Remember the movie *Apollo 13* with Tom Hanks? In April 1970, as it was heading to the moon, Apollo 13 was damaged by the explosion of one of the oxygen tanks. It was not technology that brought the Apollo spacecraft to a successful return. This kind of problem could not have been foreseen by any simulation. It was human creativity, inventiveness, and a good dose of problem solving that brought the astronauts safely back to earth.

• Medical science will never be possible without a human component. Hippocrates said that "wherever the art of medicine is loved, there is also a love of humanity." Medical science has no chance of succeeding without a smile, without the much needed pat on the back, or without the words "we're doing all that we can, it will be all right." In these times of sophisticated heart-lung machines and blinking prostheses we tend to forget this, but we all know that empathy is one of the most important catalysts of post-op recovery.

So no, we can't do without people in the operating room. We need people. People bring in creativity, gut feeling, wit, problem solving, empathy, and much more of the good stuff. But with this comes the less attractive characteristics of these creatures we call humans: thoughtlessness, overconfidence, fatigue, anxiety, disputes and stubbornness. Nothing we can do about it – it's a one-package deal. If we want to see John walking again, we can only try to utilize the good qualities and watch out for the bad.

2. PERSONAL PERFORMANCE: YOU AND YOUR BODY

—⁕—

Listen When Your Body Talks

If you asked me what is the most fascinating characteristic of the human body, I would have to say it's flexibility. The human body can function in the Sahara Desert and on the North Pole. At sea level and in the mountains. We can eat plants and we can live on meat. We lived as nomadic hunters in the north of Africa before we settled and domesticated animals. After that, we started to live in cities. The human body can keep up with it all.

However, every system has its limits. The flexibility of the human body is not infinite. To allow your body to stay in balance, you need to continually connect to it and take care of it. And for that you need time, energy and attention.

Nowadays, however, a lot of time, energy and attention is spent on activities that occur outside our bodies.

Sure, the information age has made our lives much easier. On the other hand, what was referred to fifteen years ago as "multitasking" has become normal life. The information that one had to process in a week in the Middle Ages is what we now have to swallow in an evening of web surfing. There are many things in our environment that demand our attention, and this has led to a certain detachment. We are so occupied with our outside world that we have lost connection with our bodies.

It's a simple equation – the attention and energy we give to the outside world cannot also be spent on connecting with our inner world.

We have lost track of our bodies. We ignore signals of fatigue, we ignore signals of disease, we ignore signals of indigestion. Think about animals that are not feeling well. What do they do? They lay down. They sleep for forty-eight hours until they are better. What do we do? We load ourselves up with ibuprofen and go to work. And we misinterpret our body, causing psycho-somatic illnesses. I see this every day in my practice. People with visual problems just because they don't know what their body is telling them. In our low vision department we treat people who are functionally blind, and this can be caused by mental stress or other problems in their life. Sometimes all the tests show that there is really nothing wrong with their visual system. It's possible for people to be so disconnected from their body they cannot use their visual system any more, while having a perfectly good pair of eyes!

Also, we've lost track of our food. Do you want an irrefutable advice on healthy food in one sentence? Never eat something your grandmother wouldn't recognize (I count sushi as an exception). We all know that the processed food we give to our body is not okay, and on top of that we eat too much. All of us have a sedentary lifestyle. We don't need mountains of food. How many calories do we need each day? Two thousand is more than enough for women, and 2,400 for men. Yet we stuff our faces with fat unhealthy food all day long. According to the US Department of Agriculture, in 1970 the average American daily calorie intake was 2,234. By 2003 it had risen to 2,757. This is an increase of 523 calories per day, which can lead to a weight gain of *one pound every week*.

Most of us don't really know how to recognize the signals our body is sending. No wonder. The way our body works and the way our body sends us information is complicated. Even doctors and nurses have difficulties interpreting the signals their own bodies are sending them. From what I have seen over the years, most medical personnel are perfectly capable of recognizing spastic colon or chronic back pain in their patients but completely ignore the exact same symptoms in themselves.

The reason for this is the fact that nothing in medicine is absolutely consistent. There are always exceptions. And here we see one of the many mysteries of the mind at work: most people assume they themselves are the exception. That the rules of common sense count for everybody except for them. That they are always at the periphery of the Gauss curve.

Most of us think like this:

Yes, chronic back pain is related to the posture of the body while working, but not for me.

Yes, most people aren't capable of working eight hours without eating; luckily, I'm the exception.

Yes, it makes sense to go home and relax after ten hours of continuous surgery, but I'm different, I will go to that meeting of the Institutional Review Board anyway.

Yes, my patients should all stop smoking but I will live to be one hundred and twenty while smoking a pack a day.

Another thing is this: Look at the model of the microcosm. The number one priority is the outcome, the patient. Making people better. Everything inside the system is second to the health and the treatment of our patients. All the cogwheels in the microcosm – including you – have to keep on turning no matter what, because we want to cure our patients to the best of our capabilities. So when it comes to taking care of ourselves, we often feel we don't have a choice. The long days, the sleep deprivation, the unnatural body postures, the night work, the upset stomach – most of us take it for granted because we don't want to be the cogwheel that jams the system, don't we?

Let's face it: Who cares about how you feel? Who gives a damn about your swollen ankles or your neck pain? Who will worry about the fact that you need three litres of coffee to get through the day? Not too many people, right? And the people who care will probably be found at home, not in your hospital or practice. And even if people did care in your hospital, it's so extremely uncool to talk about your feelings in a hospital environment that the subject will be avoided anyway.

There is only one person who can and will ever really take care of your body and that's *you*. Yes, your patients can still remain your top priority, but that doesn't mean you shouldn't take care of yourself. Your body is an amazing piece of work, and thanks to it's flexibility it has a built-in tendency to try to stay in balance. But it can only do that if you treat it right. As a doctor, resident, or nurse, your number one concern is the wellbeing of others, but you cannot help others if you yourself are miserable. You need to take very good care of yourself.

Do you think that's a selfish statement?

Au contraire. If I were to line up ten of your colleagues and I asked you to pick the three who were feeling good on a physical level – the ones who had the most energy, who ate healthy food, and who seem to be connected very well with their own bodies – you could probably do that quite easily, couldn't you? It shows in their eyes, their skin, their posture, and their smile. Now if I showed you the same line up and ask you to pick the three that took the best care of their patients. The ones that spend more energy on every single patient, the ones that never skip through their clinical exam. Wouldn't you agree that chances are high you would pick the same three?

Consider this. In an aircraft flying at high altitude, if the air pressure suddenly drops in the cabin, oxygen masks are dropped from the compartments above the passenger's heads. The directions are clear: Before helping others, first put on your own oxygen mask. You cannot be of any use to others if you are not fully capable of functioning.

So you need to listen to your body. If your body tells you it's really time to go home after that ten hours of continuous surgery, skip the Institutional Review Board and do so.

Walk the Ridge of the Hill

For all of us, the physical and mental level at which we function fluctuates. This level is the degree to which we are "in action," both mentally and physically. Every individual has a certain amount of physical and mental alertness, which we can call "engagement." The way in which we deal with our surroundings is greatly influenced by our level of engagement, which determines how aware we are of the world and how we process new information or choose to respond to it.

You need to have insight into your engagement level in order to know how you'll cope with stress and demanding situations. If you want your body and your brain to be your allies while doing surgery you need to know how they're doing. The main problem is that most people don't have a clue. Engagement moves along a continuous scale and influences your functioning, especially if the situation is demanding. This is why the first step to managing your performance is knowing how engaged you are: there's no use for a map if you don't know your location. Engagement is a sliding scale that goes from the most relaxed state one can be in (deep relaxed wakefulness) to the most pumped-up state (panic attack). The whole scale can be divided in to seven steps:

1. Deep relaxed wakefulness: Awake but so relaxed that we are close to being asleep.

2. Relaxation: The feeling you get after a massage or a hot bath.

3. Comfort: Reading your favorite magazine in the spring sun.

4. Vigilance mode: Somewhat laid-back but still alert, not too stressed but also not too relaxed. You're smoothly engaged in everyday events.

5. Agitation: Feeling on edge, cross, stressed.

6. Hyperarousal: On top of the bungee jump platform, ankle attachment secured.

7. Panic Attack: Losing control, sense of going crazy, being in physical overdrive.

So while working in a demanding environment like an operating room, where should you ideally be on the engagement scale? What's the best physical and mental state? Well, somewhere near the halfway mark would be best. This is what we call vigilance mode, somewhat laid-back but still alert, not too stressed but also not too relaxed.

Vigilance mode is what you could to call "walking the ridge of the hill." Imagine you are on a hiking trip with a group of close friends. The weather is beautiful. The sky is blue, the sun is shining, you're all carrying backpacks, and you're enjoying the walk. After you've been traveling uphill for quite a while, the track starts to follow the ridge of a steep hill. You're enjoying the nice view, laughing and joking with your friends, but there is a little red light blinking in the back of your head telling you not to feel too comfortable. There is no need to stress out, but yet you should be careful. One false step might buy you a one-way ticket down the hillside. So there you are, right between comfort and agitation. You're in vigilance mode.

In surgery this means partially relying on calmness and routine while at the same time being fully alert and watchful. It can be a tricky balancing act. Nevertheless, if you can keep their engagement scale at vigilance mode you have three huge advantages:

First, you perform better than average. Those who are able to increase their engagement level if they are too relaxed and can tune it down if they have too much adrenaline in their blood usually do a much better job. They are both in the right physical modus and in the right frame of mind. I know, everybody is different and some people will thrive when they're really relaxed, others will when they're more on edge. But the deviation from vigilance mode at which people can be still in an optimal situation to function is limited. The way in which we can make optimal use of our body and our mind's capabilities decreases rapidly if we deviate too much from that sweet spot we call vigilance mode.

Second, the more you're in vigilance mode, the more pleasant you are to work with. Especially people who lean towards the right side of the scale can make other's blood boil. We all know them – the over-stressed surgeons. The ones who run their ortho-sympathetic nervous system in overdrive from down till dark. They run instead of walk, they shout instead of talk, and they scare the hell out of everybody around them. Just to avoid them, colleagues will skip the elevator for five floors of stairs. You don't want to be that person, do you? The thing is this: what you radiate, you will get back. The people around you work like a mirror. If you radiate agitation and frustration, you'll be surrounded by people who are likewise agitated and frustrated. If you radiate composure, kindness and confidence, you'll find yourself surrounded by cool, kind and confident people. It really is as simple as that.

Third, by being in vigilance mode, you prevent the burning of all of your energy in the first two hours of your day. Look at it this way: in the morning you get one barrel of energy. Avoiding stress is the only way to have some energy left after you've finished work. When driving home from work we sometimes feel like a squeezed orange. Not so long ago a colleague told me, "You know, when I come home after a long day of surgery, I park my car in the drive and I walk towards the front door. When I am at the door, I hear my children playing and shouting inside the house. I know that they will be so glad to see me, the second I open the door they will be pouncing on top of me. That's a wonderful feeling. But sometimes I feel so tired, I really wish I had some more energy left for the evenings. For my children, for my wife, for my hobbies. Sometimes it's really a tall order to hitch up my pants, grab the doorknob and say let's go."

Routine Can Be Your Best Friend

When talking about the engagement scale, one side of this scale is characterized by relaxation or being laid-back. In relation to performance, this is typically the moment when routine kicks in. The more we feel at ease, the more we start to rely on routine. Being more relaxed means that it's easy to continue what you're doing and that you don't need to rely on sheer willpower to persevere. The more relaxed you are, the more you'll be be storing energy for later on. If you're relaxed, you can work from habit, relying on routine instead of deliberation. This is a good thing, because you cannot think of everything all the time anyway; perfectly micro-managing your performance is impossible. Working from habit means that you do things the way in which you've learnt to do them throughout your years of experience.

You'll be more sociable if you're relaxed. Feeling comfortable is one of the greatest things you can do for your colleagues and the people who are around you during work. You'll be pleasant to work with and will contribute more to any team effort. It's hard to work with stressed-out, irritable people! You'll be in control of your own body. There's nothing like a pounding heart or shaky hands to make you feel like you're the victim of circumstances. Relaxation means you can confidently take matters in your own hands. It will also allow you to widen your field of view and see things in perspective.

This is efficient, but it comes with the danger of inattention. In other words, routine is both your best friend and your enemy. As your proverbial field of view widens, the size of your blind spot will unfortunately also increase. Your physical blind spot is that part of the retina (the cells at the back of your eyes) where the optic nerve is attached to carry signals to the brain. This blind spot is located just to the side of the macula, which is the exact center of your vision and which has the highest acuity. The funny thing about your blind spot is that you virtually never notice it. There's a blank spot in your vision, but you're not aware of it because your brain fills in the missing information!

Things can happen right in front of our nose without us noticing.

Too much relaxation can cause you to take things too lightly. Once they're relaxed, people tend to lean back and crack jokes. There's nothing wrong with that *per se*, but you need to remember that any time spent on small talk is not being put to the task at hand. Humans become overconfident about the future if they are too relaxed. If things are running smoothly, we tend to believe they will continue doing so. If things are going well, we stop questioning our assumptions.

As a consequence, we slack off a bit, fully convinced things will turn out right anyway. Once we notice any negligence it may already be too late.

Whatever we do, there are always some things that we're taking for granted but which should be met with a healthy dose of skepticism. This skepticism should work like a background scanner, constantly reviewing all the assumptions we're making. Whether you're assuming that certain things will happen, that people will act in a certain way, or that equipment will actually work, you need to stay aware of the fact that reality has a way of turning out differently. While it's impossible to evaluate and double check each and every thing, you should definitely stay alert and look whether your assumptions hold. Any relaxed atmosphere is labile – and dangerously so! A small setback may be more than relaxed people can handle. Once routine fails, they may break into a frenzy, stress out, and cause more mistakes because they're overcome with doubt. So, yes, being relaxed makes us feel good, which in turn makes us work smoothly and amiably. However, this comes at the risk of being too nonchalant and error-prone, which can make mistakes spiral out of control.

So be ware of routine. Watch out for unthinking routine in your own actions and those of your team. In my experience, the best way to avoid too much routine is to now and then deliberately break the routine.

The first thing to do is to be aware that things are running smoothly – perhaps too smoothly. When you notice that everybody is running too much on routine, stir things up a little. Talk about what could happen. Make a strong point about something. Ask some questions to bring everybody back in to focus. As they say, you need to flutter the dovecotes (for my American readers, shake things up) a bit once in a while. Some airline companies deliberately mix the crews to make sure that people don't get too accustomed to the same team. By making sure people cannot fly with the same cockpit crew for more than three flights in a row, they brake habits and avoid routine. The same can be done in the OR. As much as you like to work with your trusted scrub nurse who has been with you for fifteen years, it's a good idea to ask someone ask to scrub in from time to time.

What to Do When Adrenalin Gets the Better of You

Being agitated is not a bad thing by itself. It's nothing more than leaning towards the agitated part of the engagement scale; and since the adrenalin in your bloodstream brings your whole body in action mode, you'll be more alert and attentive. You'll scan your environment, looking for flaws and errors. You'll be more critical towards yourself and others. You'll not assume too much, but you'll be skeptical and will double (or triple) check everything. You'll be ready to act.

Engagement causes bodily changes to happen, which will allow you to react more quickly if necessary. More blood will flow to your muscles and your posture will change. You'll be more focused. Adrenaline narrows your field of view and makes you attend solely to the task at hand. Distractions in the environment are filtered out when you're engaged. So when your orthosympathetic nervous system shifts into fifth gear, that's not necessarily a bad thing. The key is to know the advantages and the risks.

The signals that your body sends you when an overdose of adrenalin flows through your veins are the same signals you would receive when you're standing on top of the Royal Gorge Bridge in Colorado, a thick bungee rope around your ankles, ready to jump:

- Your heart is racing like a Harley engine at full throttle.
- Your breathing is fast and shallow.
- Your hands are shaking.

- Your neck is hot.

- You feel sweaty, nauseous, and dizzy.

- Your hands and legs may seem to have a will of their own.

The problem is that when adrenalin kicks in, most people are usually not planning to jump off a bridge. They're about to give a piano recital. They're waiting for their turn to give a speech at their brother's wedding. They're about to make an important presentation at work. They're negotiating with their boss about their pension plan.

Or, as in your case, they might be draping the patient, getting ready to start a shoulder arthroscopy.

In all these cases, our body fails at the moment we need it the most. When you think of it, it's strange that a system that was developed to respond in the most critical moments in our lives burdens us with a ton of symptoms that make even breathing difficult, let alone creating a watertight vascular anastomosis with a 6/0 polypropylene suture. Sure enough, when your two-year-old daughter all of a sudden darts into the street, it's adrenalin that enables you to grab her by the arm in a split second. The same is true in experiences like escaping burning buildings, jumping away from falling rocks, or getting to a safe spot when a gorilla escapes from the zoo.

But how often do such things happen? Almost never, right? Still, we need the sympathetic nervous system. As with all alarm systems, sometimes all signals need to turn red, however small the odds of this happening may be. (Ask the woman who was attacked in 2007 in the zoo in Rotterdam by an escaped gorilla named Bokito.) The problem is that the sympathetic nervous system doesn't turn on only when real problems occur. Activation of the system is not preceded by a logical or rational estimation of the possible danger. There is no buffer that causes you to consider whether or not it would be useful to activate your body's turbo. There's no time for that when your two-year-old is about to be run over by a car. That's why activation of this system happens very fast and is reactive. It doesn't take much to activate it. This system is trigger happy!

However, the tremor and the pounding heartbeat is just one part of the problem. There is one big misconception about tremor, and that is that you cannot operate when you have it. This is not true. Even in the field of microsurgery, which I happen to know quite well, it's possible to do a good job while having a tremor. I have witnessed many surgeons doing an excellent job while having a certain degree of tremor. It might well be the biggest taboo in surgery. Nobody likes to talk about it, and in my opinion most of us consider it a big deal. It's not. A bit of shaky hands is not a big deal and it won't put an end to your brilliant surgical career!

The main problem with adrenalin is not the bodily reactions but the fact that it paralyzes your brain. Stress will put your body in survival mode, which means that more blood will be sent to base brain regions such as the brainstem. Less blood will be sent to your prefrontal cortex, where much of our logical thought and deliberation takes place. As stress hormones change the state of your brain, you'll find yourself less capable of thinking in a structured manner. Dr. Clifton K. Meador once said, "It's usually the second mistake in response to the first that does the patient in," and indeed, this is often the case. When things get difficult it's the absence of the normal, logical reasoning that we normally rely on that causes the problem to turn in to a disaster. The first event throws us out of our comfort zone and our reaction to that might be something we often refer to starting with, "What was I thinking when I…"

So, all right. At a certain moment, for one reason or another, adrenalin gets the better of us. And what do we do? When something happens that we don't like, we start fighting it. We try to come to grips with the issue and are determined to deal with the problem. No such luck. Not only is it a completely unfair fight, it's one you definitely don't want to fight. Because the more you fight the symptoms of adrenalin, the worse they become. The more convulsively you try to control your body, the more difficult this becomes.

Here's the catch. The title of this book is misleading. In the operating room, there is plenty of room for shaky hands. The question is what is your reaction to the shaky hands. If you can avoid to try to control the shaky hands you will be fine. If you start to fight things will only get worse. There is only one real solution: observe and accept. Stop fighting! Become both the observer and acceptor of what you're feeling. No fighting. No judging. No trying to change things. Better still, the more comfortable you become with observing and accepting, the easier it gets.

It's an Aikido thing. Morihei Ueshiba, the founder of Aikido said, "There are no contests in Aikido. A true warrior is invincible because he or she contests with nothing. Defeat means to defeat the mind of contention that we harbor within." The key is to not confront your opponent head on but to use his force against himself. It's completely unnatural and it's 100% counter-intuitive, but it's the only way.

You know that surgeons have a mindset of "take action and fix the damn problem!" And especially for action minded people, learning to *do* things is much easier then learning what *not* to do. But it's possible. Each time adrenalin pops up, try to take a step back, detach yourself from the situation, so to speak, and watch what happens like an observer.

At some point, you'll be able to encourage the symptoms. You'll say, "If we have to go through this, let's get it over with! Come on, is this the best you can do? Bring it on!"

Excellent!

But wait a minute. When I'm in a situation where I feel dizzy and nauseous, do I need to ask to have more stress added to the situation? Sweat is pouring down my back, my legs are shaking, and I'm supposed to ask, "Is this the best you can do?"

Yes. That is exactly what I'm saying. Fear feeds on fear, you know. The moment you're thinking, "I hope this doesn't get worse," you're fighting fire with fire. You're just adding more worry and uncertainty to the situation, which only makes you feel worse.

The moment you think "Bring it on," you put out the fire, however illogical that may sound. It works fantastically. Your fears, rapid heartbeats, and shaking hands will melt away.

Be Fit to Fly

First of all, let me say this. I'm going to discuss sleep deprivation, and I know what you're thinking. Ophthalmologists have no right to talk about sleep deprivation. Really. We have no idea what it's like to be called into an acute appendicitis in the middle of the night, let alone face one for the third night in a row. We don't know how it feels to head into fourteen hours of surgery after a mere two hours of sleep. As far as sleep deprivation goes, ophthalmologists are wimps. With the exception of the occasional trauma, we usually spend our nights in slumberland. I'm fine with that, as I happen to like my bed a lot.

Somebody who does know what he's talking about on the subject of sleep deprivation is Professor Czeisler from the Harvard Medical School. He and his colleagues have done extensive research into the effects of sleep deprivation on the performance of medical residents. The results are shocking. Residents running more than five marathon shifts a month (i.e., shifts of more than twenty-four hours each) did not just show an increased amount of medical mistakes; they were also confronted with a significant increase of their patient mortality. Moreover, the residents themselves were at an increased risk of car accidents. Doctors without sleep are not just a danger to their patients, but also to themselves!

Unfortunately, sleep deprivation is part of medical culture, especially among surgeons. There is some sort of heroism surrounding lack of sleep: just picture the indefatigable surgeon who is able to save lives in the middle of the night, only to fix himself up with three cups of coffee at dawn before he proceeds with another day of elective surgery. A true hero, right? Not really. Research shows that patients should really try to avoid this type of surgeon. Odds of hemorrhages, organ injuries, wound failures, and other problems nearly double if the surgeon skips a night. This is also true for routine cases!

You might wonder why hospitals do not solve this problem. I do, too. The most often-heard argument is an economical one: if people work less, costs will increase. The reasoning is that limiting the hours a surgeon makes would force the hiring of more surgeons, leading to additional costs.

While this point is true, the argument as a whole may not hold water. Add the costs of treating the complications of poor surgery, such as staff costs and resources, and the economics will definitely change.

Besides, costs should not be the only argument. Would you agree to be operated on by someone who has been awake for twenty-four hours, in the knowledge that this boosts the odds of all sorts of complications, including death? Would you allow a family member to be treated that way? I am sure even the financial manager of your hospital would answer both questions with a negative.

Sure, I can hear you think, "I understand what you're saying, but I'm not in control of my hours. I'm part of a system that I cannot change. My hands are tied – if I were up all night performing surgery and were called to operate in the morning, I cannot change that. It's just the way things work."

You're right, of course. Changing the system is hard and will take a lot of time. But there are some things you can do.

First of all, you can be aware of the problem. This is an important step! Know that sleep deprivation affects your cognition and your actions. Know that it weakens your attention, leads to brain fog, and makes you less aware of what's happening around you.

Sleep deprivation also affects your decision-making capacity. If you're low on sleep, you'll often become a little too expeditious, according to research. Drastic decisions are easily made under sleep-deprived circumstances, probably just to get things over with and go to bed!

On the other end of the spectrum, severe lethargy can also lead to indecisiveness. Weighing pros and cons is a lot harder if you're tired. Once you realize that poor sleep can greatly affect your response to the environment, you've come a long way.

If you're tired, the second thing you can do is look for replacements. It may be that somebody else can take over your job in the OR. This is especially true if you're a resident – is there any place in the hospital that residents like more than the OR? Sure, it will probably mean you yourself will have to move to a place that you like a little bit less, like the outpatient clinic. But hey, the main goal of hospitals is not to make *you* as happy as possible. It's to improve the health of *patients*.

A third option is to postpone surgery. This is a grand taboo, and you're probably coming up with all sorts of objections right now, but bear with me. Let's imagine that you've been up all night, performing surgery on a multi-trauma patient. You have another case scheduled at 7:45 AM – a revision of a hip prosthesis – and none of your colleagues has the skills to fill in for you. So, you'll have to make do with two hours of sleep.

Consider this alternative: if you postpone the surgery to 9:45 AM, you can double your amount of sleep. But your gut reaction is now telling you that this is impossible. Who postpones surgery? You have a patient who is prepared for a certain time, you have a team ready for surgery, and leaving the OR empty is a waste of money! If you postpone, you'll be chastised by your medical chief! Also, you'd finish later in the afternoon and miss that game of tennis you were looking forward to! It just can't happen!

And that's where you're wrong. All of the above objections are real arguments, but none of them makes postponing a physical impossibility. In fact, if a power failure occurred, you'd also postpone. So while it may be awkward, inappropriate, stupid, and expensive on the short run, it's possible to reschedule surgery. I'm not saying it's easy. It's just not impossible.

The fourth and final way to contribute to a less sleep-deprived hospital is by taking a stand each time work hours or sleep-deprivation become the topic of discussion. Statistical evidence is mounting and it's time we face the facts: sleep-deprived surgeons are crappy surgeons.

We'll need to keep repeating this message to make sure everybody gets it. Only then can we see gradual change on all levels: among surgeons and staff, among management and human resource departments, among politicians and educators. Now, I may sound like a politician looking to spread his grand message, but I'm dead serious here. Each time work hours are discussed, always take the side of research and common sense. Truck drivers need to take regular breaks by law. They have tachographs mounted to their vehicles to ensure that. So why shouldn't doctors follow sleep patterns that can literally save lives?

In aviation they use the phrase "fit to fly." If a pilot doesn't feel well due to sickness, extreme fatigue, or other causes, he or she can call in and say they're not fit to fly. The airline company then looks for replacement. For surgeons, I believe we also owe it to our patients to confess when we're really not fit to fly, and look for replacement. I know this is not always possible. If the helicopter with the liver transplant has already landed on the roof of your hospital and you're the only hepatic surgeon around, you might still be the patient's best bet, sick or not. But as far as possible, everybody who sets foot in the operating room should be fit to fly.

Know Your Weak Spots

Some years ago I attended a lecture by a group of research-ers who had investigated the incidence of complications during surgery. Instead of taking the usual approach and grouping their data by surgeon or by some pre-operative factor, they looked at their data in a clever, novel way: they plotted the amount of com-plications that occurred in their hospital as a function of time of day. The resulting graph illustrated how the rate of complica-tions changed during the day.

This made for an interesting picture. At 8:00 AM, compli-cation rates were moderate. Between 9:00 and 10:00 AM they declined to their lowest rate. This makes sense, as people need some time to warm up. At about 10:30 AM, when surgery had been going on for more than two hours and staff was getting tired and hypoglycemic, complications showed a huge spike. After the 11:00 AM coffee break, the risk of complications low-ered to a steady level for the rest of the day. This surprised me, as I had expected the post-lunch dip to cause at least a bit of an increase.

In any case, if I'd ever need cataract surgery myself, I know I'd like to be scheduled at 9:00 AM!

However, we shouldn't generalize these findings, since the complication rate involves a lot of variables. It may depend a variety of factors including the type of surgery, on the number of surgeons in the operating room, and the individual and col-lective experience of the team. Your own individual graph might look wholly different. Some people perform best in the morning while others peak in the afternoon. Doing surgery at 9:00 AM is no surefire way to guarantee success for everyone!

The lesson to draw here is that your performance will fluctuate during the day. Make sure you know your own strengths and weaknesses. Identify your periods of peak performance. While fatigue and hypoglycemia change over the course of the day, you'll find there are day-to-day patterns for you as an individual. For example, I know I work best for periods of two hours with intermittent breaks. I also know I need to take care if I get hungry around 4:00 PM, because otherwise my focus will slip away.

Knowing yourself enables you to anticipate a decreased level of functioning. Keep a log of complications and resurgeries, and make sure you add all details: what surgery, what time, which OR, and which instruments. Surgeons who maintain an accurate database of their performance can reach fascinating insights. I know one surgeon who meticulously records his work and found out his success rate for one particular procedure was higher for left eyes than for right eyes! If you know when you're at your best, you can schedule your work optimally. Are you someone who needs a little time before you're on a roll? Make sure you start your day with a procedure you're really good at and do the more difficult cases after that. If you know that you peak around 2:00 PM, make sure you plan your most challenging surgery around that time.

Similarly, knowing your own weaknesses helps. Some of them may be remedied by training or education. Others may simply be a part of you. If you've always needed nine hours of sleep to be fully rested, it doesn't make any sense to try and change that.

Instead, you should organize your life in a way that accommodates the way you are.

In all microcosms where excellent human performance is required, one of the main questions is this: should people try to improve their weaknesses or should they accept them and work around them?

The answer is tricky. I have seen people work on their weaknesses and get great joy out of that. There is nothing more fulfilling then getting a bit better every day and improving who you are and what you're capable of. Here's a personal example. For most of my adult life I was never good with computers and I certainly took no notice whatsoever of the technology with which websites are built. But I recently decided that I wanted to change that because this book would benefit from a promotional website, and if I had built the site myself I would be much more flexible in changing the content. So I sank my teeth into it and a couple of weeks later *voilà* , there it was.

So I would say work on your weaker skills either if you can get joy out of that or if you need them to do things only you can do – things that cannot be outsourced.

However, from what I have seen it is often a good idea to work with your strengths and around your weaknesses. The people I know to be highly efficient at what they do have a crystal clear idea of what their weaknesses are and how to avoid needing to rely on them.

You'll need to make up your own mind. The answer is within you and only you know which talents you have and which skills ought to be improved.

Take operating time, for example. You might be like me and perform better while doing relatively short surgeries that take between twenty minutes and two hours. It definitely played a role in my decision to specialize in surgery of the anterior part of the eye and not to opt for the long procedures of retinal surgery, the back of the eye. Who could give advice on that? Nobody. One person might say long surgeries are hard, another may find them boring and a third person may think they are fantastic. Ask the same question to a thousand people and you'll get a thousand answers. You'll have to make up your own mind.

Manage Your Energy

Each morning, as our alarms wake us, we get one bucket of energy to get us through the day. Some people use their energy responsibly and are able to work all a day and then go out for a game of golf in the evening. Others already have an empty bucket by midday and need to pull themselves through the afternoon, only to end up in front of some mindless sitcom on TV. It pays off to manage your energy well, even though doing so can be tricky.

Managing your energy is not only about getting to that golf course. Compared to other occupations, surgery leaves little room for error. Patients expect high performance and surgeons want to do the best job they can, each time around. This means that every time you walk into the OR you need to have the energy to strive for perfection. If you don't, you shouldn't attempt it. For every single task that is on your to-do list you should ask yourself, "Am I going to do this or not?" For every task that you set aside there are two other possibilities: you either have someone else do it or it doesn't get done at all.

The first option – have someone else do it – is quite common in the corporate sector. If you don't have time to do it, outsource it! In surgery, this outsourcing of work is much more difficult. In fact it's likely that only a small part of your job can delegated to others because only you can do the work you do. While this situation is not ideal, for many surgeons it's simply the reality. Still, if possible, you should have somebody else do those tasks you're not up for. In the end, this is in everyone's best interest including yours and, more importantly, your patient's.

The second option – it doesn't get done at all – is especially relevant for tasks that serve no immediate purpose to you or maybe even no purpose at all! "No" is an important word in the vocabulary of excellent surgeons. Why go to a useless weekly meeting if this means missing the grand rounds? Why read that forty-page report that is wholly unconnected to your department? Why fill in thirty-year-old forms, for which no one can even guess the purpose? Make sure you always consider how useful a task is, and to what extent it adds to your only real task – treating patients well.

You need to balance your energy within the complex dynamics of a hospital. Yes, the quality of patient care, the amount of treatments, finances, the training of residents and fellows, the reception of guests, safety rules and regulations, and countless other issues are of great importance. But like everyone else, you woke up with that single bucket of energy! First and foremost, you need to focus on those tasks that are relevant to your core business: being an excellent surgeon. If that involves delegating tasks to someone else or leaving them altogether, so be it.

The same thing goes for giving your opinion. If someone wants to know your thoughts about a broken coffee machine or about the new manager of a distant hospital while you're busy, there's no shame in telling them it's not of interest to you.

Over the last thirty years many books have been written about time management. The problem with time management is that for a surgeon, time management has its limits. A procedure that was scheduled to take one hour can suddenly become a four-hour job. And since a lot of work we do is one-on-one, a significant part of our time is filled with fixed, defined activities.

Energy management is different.

First of all, you need to use your energy sparingly; but the nice thing is that it can be created by doing things you love. Every single one of us has stuff they genuinely like to do during the day. These are things that are close to our hearts and things that let us forget time. Yes, also in our job! Focus on those activities and you'll create energy. The saving of energy won't be so much of an issue anymore because you'll have plenty.

So use and manage your energy wisely. Of course, priorities change throughout the day. If there is little surgery going on, you can safely invest energy in training, or discuss issues not directly related to your work. If you're mentally rehearsing scenarios for a difficult procedure, and you're fully occupied by preparing this surgery, it's perfectly okay to duck that talkative intern. Life is all about making the right decisions, and sometimes that might be hiding from someone who eats away your time and energy.

Just don't get caught hiding behind the x-ray machine. It's such a silly sight.

Here's my rule to remember: *The things that are important must never be at the mercy of the things that matter less.*

In other words, concentration and attention have two sides. On one hand you have the *focusing* on one particular task. Your ability to focus and to concentrate directly affects the results of your surgery.

And on the other hand there is the *avoidance of distraction.*

In the operating room you're aware of a world of events. The residents talking, a medicine that is drawn into a syringe from a flask, the scrubbing nurse who's looking for her favorite station on the radio, the anesthetist who's going through the medical file of the patient – all of it's going on around you. But that doesn't mean that you know what's going on around you. Most people have the tendency to think that we're reasonably aware of what's going on around us. We think that we get most of the information trough our senses and that the things we don't see, hear, smell, taste, or feel are picked up in some way trough a mysterious sixth sense.

The reality is different. Imaging that you're in a dark room with a flashlight in your hand. You turn the flashlight on and shine it directly ahead. Everything that is hit by the bundle of light bears information about what is in the room. All the rest is there but you can't see it because the flashlight is not directed towards it. This is the same for your attention in the operating room.

One of the most important founders of the American philosophy, William James, wrote, "Attention is the taking possession of the mind, in clear and vivid form, of one out of what may seem several simultaneously possible objects or trains of thoughts. It implies withdrawal from some things to deal effectively with others." Take a moment to look at what's going on around you while you read this text. Look around and listen. Do you hear birds chirping? A train in the distance? Is the cat purring a couple of yards away? Because all your attention was focused on the text in this book, you may have had a vague awareness of these things but no specific interest in them.

3. PERSONAL PERFORMANCE: YOU AND YOUR MIND

—⚏—

A Flashlight in the Dark

The reason you need to know where your attention is going is that during surgery, you really need to stay focused on the job. You need to be aware of everything that's relevant to the procedure. No more, no less. You can view the OR as a recurrent interaction between people and environment, with a constant flow between:

1. Reality. Everything that happens around you and which you could perceive.

2. Observation. The information that reaches your senses and is perceived by you. (Blood saturation, systolic blood pressure, operating time.)

3. Analysis. Processing this information and comparing it to knowledge and past experience. (How much time left before CO_2 levels will start to rise.)

4. Decision. Considering potential actions, making the right decision. (Let's abandon the laparoscopy and open up the patient.)

5. Action. Turning your decision into action, which then becomes a part of reality, thus closing the cycle. (Ten blade, please.)

A large part of surgery is getting into this flow and continuously cycling through the steps of this reality-action cycle. Still, if you do, the question remains what information really reaches you. There are many things to look at, but you don't consciously perceive them all. Like a great filter, your focused attention selectively allows some information to get through while halting the rest. Like a flashlight in the dark, attention highlights just a specific part of the world.

Research has shown that medical mistakes are often due to surgeons not getting certain information. Pointing the flashlight in the wrong direction – or perhaps having too weak a flashlight – they fail at step 2, and therefore at all subsequent steps! If your attention is not focused, due to lack of energy or other circumstances, you're at risk of performing poorly.

As an illustration, consider the following anecdote by an anesthesiologist I recently talked to. "I was with a patient during a knee prosthesis procedure, when my OR manager came in with a question about a form that I had supposedly filled in one day earlier. She had found two mistakes in the form and wanted to talk about them. I looked at the form and was surprised to see that the form showed my name and the numbers were in my handwriting, but I really couldn't remember having filled it in. The manager insisted that I had and I got a bit annoyed, especially since the form contained errors and I always take care to be accurate with such things.

"To check the handwriting, I went to a pile of documents stacked in the corner. Then I heard a voice calling out my name. 'This is the third time I've called you – what's wrong with you,?' the voice said. 'Your machine is making terrible noises, shut it down!'

"Only then did I realize an alarm was ringing. One of the tubes had gotten kinked and the patient was receiving poor ventilation! None of this had gotten through to me. I was so focused on the documents that I hadn't noticed any of the sounds."

This story shows how limited our perception of the world can be. Always make sure you point the flashlight in the right direction, with the right intensity! You don't want to miss anything important.

Attention Thieves Are Everywhere

One day I was with a colleague who was performing cataract operations. It was crowded in the OR – there were people who were busy with cables, flat-screens, video cameras, and recording equipment. As it turned out a new video recording system was being tested with which 3D recordings could be made. The immense black flat-screen TV that was standing on a shiny metal table was the latest model 3D television. And I thought that those things only were sold to watch 3D movies at home! Two high-definition cameras were connected to the microscope and together registered a three-dimensional image that was run through a tower of expensive digital boxes on the 3D TV.

Sitting behind the operating microscope, with the patient already covered for the operation, the surgeon greeted me with two pairs of glasses perched on his nose. One pair of glasses was his regular pair, and on top of that he wore a different pair of specially polarized 3D glasses. It was just like watching a 3D animation at the movies nowadays. The three people from the firm that came to install the recording equipment were busy running around while, full of enthusiasm, my colleague started the operation. He muttered something about the 3D glasses that somewhat hindered his image but what could go wrong? He already had performed thousands of cataract operations! And besides, only by wearing the 3D glasses could he now and then look on the monitor to admire the 3D effect of the two cameras that were mounted on the microscope.

Sure enough, it didn't take long before things went wrong. One of the most feared complications arose – a rupture of the lens capsule. That actually means that the capsule in which the lens is held breaks so that the lens falls back into the eye. Bad stuff. "That's odd," my colleague said as he looked me straight in the eye through the grayish shiny lenses of the 3D glasses. "It's been years since I've had this complication. I really have no idea what could have been the cause of it."

Of course not! Because he was looking straight through them, he couldn't see that the cause of the problem was the 3D glasses!

The reason why I love this story is the fact that it shows how easily we're tempted to let things interfere with our attention. In the operating room, when gimmicks, visitors, and technology are asking for a piece of our attention, it's sometimes very difficult to say "no." Especially when we're doing "routine" surgery, some of us are glad that there are some distractions to play around with. There is nothing wrong with having a bit at fun during these boring cases, isn't it? So when we're lured into engaging in a mindless discussion about basketball, or answering intrusive questions about some forms that have nothing to do with the procedure at hand, we don't resist. Instead we're even glad that these distractions came along to spice things up a bit. The song on the radio that we particularly like, the nice interns that are visiting the OR, that new high definition video recorder – we're attracted like magnets to things like that. It's so very difficult to resist the temptation, especially when we're doing routine cases and we think we can get away with it.

Like my colleague who had no clue whatsoever about what was limiting his visibility, often we aren't aware of the problem. Attention thieves are everywhere, and sometimes they're hard to avoid. For example, I'm used to having interns and medical students in the OR for training, but sometimes it can be hard to teach them because I'm occupied with the surgery. It took me a while to come up with a solution for that, because in the end, visitors are here to learn; and to learn from surgery, somebody needs to explain to them what the surgery is about. One day I had this genial brain wave. I said to the resident who saw assisting me, "You know, you're one of the cleverest residents I've ever had with me in the OR. You've got it all figured out. You know exactly what I'm doing. Why don't *you* explain to these nice interns what I'm doing here."

Brilliant, isn't it? Everybody was happy. The interns got the teaching that they came for, the resident felt like a champ, and I could focus on the surgery. Sometimes you need to be creative. The chance of complications increases when you direct your attention on things that distract you (three mildly sweating technicians dancing around a 3D TV monitor, just to name one of them).

Do One Thing and Do It Well

One of the most pervasive myths of our time is the myth of multitasking. Maybe it's the information overload we experience on a daily basis. There are so many things in the world that vie for our attention that our consciousness becomes fragmented. No wonder people tell themselves that they can process all incoming information at the same time. After all, there is no way to deal with all these impulses one by one!

Whatever our reasons for believing in it, research shows that true multitasking hardly exists. We can combine automated tasks (walking) with conscious tasks (talking), we can sometimes combine tasks that draw on different regions of the brain (tapping to a beat on the radio and reading the newspaper), but we certainly cannot perform comparable tasks simultaneously. People who seem like they can do this are just very adept at rapid switching between tasks. This is why multitasking is sometimes called "switchtasking" instead.

However, switching between tasks almost always causes a loss of productivity and/or quality. This loss becomes bigger if the tasks at hand require you to continuously update the current state of the problem in your mind. In other words, if a task strongly depends on the reality-action cycle mentioned before, it isn't suitable for switchtasking, even if you're good at it! As surgery requires a focused mind that is continuously prepared to pick up any relevant, odd signals and to quickly turn them into action, it's not wise to combine it with other tasks. And why should you? If the multitasking challenge of using a cell phone while driving is deemed too dangerous, why would you try to combine two, three, or even four activities in the OR?

When it comes to multitasking, there's a big difference between what we *think* we do and what we *actually* do. Let's say we want to do task A and task B simultaneously. And let's presume the maximal quality of each performed tasks is one hundred percent. What do we think we do? We think that when we perform A and B at the same time, each is performed at one hundred percent.

What is the reality? We do task A at 70%, while B is running in the background at thirty percent. Then we switch to task B, which is then at 70% and task A is performed at a lousy thirty percent. And so we switch between A and B, creating the illusion that we're doing A and B at the same time and convincing ourselves that we are doing a great job.

You know, people who are considered to be good multitaskers are just fast switchers.

So, choose one single task to focus on in the OR (so why not pick surgery, just to name one example), and don't also try to keep several conversations going or to plan for an upcoming meeting. You should feel free to communicate, of course – there's no reason to completely avoid small talk in the OR. But keep in mind that the best surgeons are those who keep surgery prioritized at all times. Only when it's completed, can we have our minds enter the mode of another task.

Pick Up the Blade for Real

Surgery can be a real challenge. There are cases where potential complications are overwhelming. However, you should always make that first incision with determination and a sense of purpose. A neurosurgeon friend once told me, "When I'm dealing with a really challenging case, such as an aneurysm that's hard to reach, I find that there's a linear relationship between the difficulty and my confidence. The less certain I am about the outcome of the intervention, the more I have a sense of firmness and a determination to give it my best shot. The less control I have over the 'what,' the more I feel my control over the 'how.' And isn't the question of how we handle things in the OR just as important as the question of what happens?"

He's right. There is no room for aimlessness in surgery. Even if you don't know exactly what to expect and cannot devise a foolproof plan of action, you still need to feel that you'll do all that is possible to make the procedure work. If you point the tip of the blade towards the disinfected skin of your patient, you should be convinced that you can deal with any problems and technical challenges that may occur! No matter the situation, the aim of your work should always be clear: improve the health of your patient. You need to be convinced that you can and will make that happen. And even if you run into problems that can't be fixed, make sure you can look back afterwards knowing that you did what you could. You came as prepared as one could be and you ran into problems that nobody could have managed. Bad luck happens. The thing is, as long as you stand tall and engage with confidence, you're most likely going to overcome any problem.

It's when you're doubtful that the battle is already lost before it has begun.

This is also true for routine surgeries. In fact, these are when you need to take special care, as it's easy to let things slide during "easier" procedures. Surgery is a challenging occupation. A sales representative can have a few bad days as long as his monthly average success rate is good. Surgery is different. As much as we like to look at the statistics, complication rates, and numbers, we all know that the patient who is on the operating table doesn't care about the statistics. And that's a difficult contradiction. Every surgeon understands the need to do things right each and every time, while knowing this is not possible. For the patient who puts his life in your hands, things need to be right this time, right now. He won't really care about your impressive average if he has to suffer through a complicated surgery.

When you pick up the blade, pick it up firmly. Pick it up for real.

Your Mind Is a Player

Your mind guides your body. It helps you choose the proper course of action at all times, so that you (ideally) avoid harm and find pleasure. The mind stays at its job all the time: observing, analyzing, judging. Even when you aren't speaking, your mind is rattling. Even if nothing really exciting is happening around you, your mind wanders and starts fantasizing and contemplating. Human beings seem to be permanently tuned into their own radio station: chatterbox FM.

Now, the programming of chatterbox FM is not entirely balanced. While the mind judges all incoming information and determines whether it's novel or expected, whether it's useful or dangerous, and whether it calls for action or dismissal, it's especially tuned to potential danger. This makes some evolutionary sense: it's a real shame to miss out on a tasty piece of fruit, but it's a much bigger problem if you miss that poisonous shake hissing in the bushes. In this regard, chatterbox FM is a bit like the news: it's biased towards the negative side of things!

When you're facing external challenges, it's a bit like playing a game. Your opponents are the circumstances and the difficulty level of the surgery. You must face them no matter how they come. A routine carpal tunnel surgery, on a patient who is comfortably under general anaesthesia, with the most experienced scrub nurse at your side, should be a smooth undertaking – a piece of cake. A difficult case of endometriosis on a patient with hemodynamic instability, surrounded by residents and nurses who have hardly ever seen the inside of an OR, is what we call a tough nut to crack.

The internal challenge, however, is of a different kind. When chatterbox FM reminds us of all the things that can go wrong, it can also be informative and help us prepare to meet external challenges. But if thoughts about possible negative outcomes become too strong, these thoughts themselves turn into opponents. We then become our own worst enemies!

Obstacles like self-doubt, nervousness, and fear are tremendously hard to overcome, exactly because they come from inside your own mind. Let's take self-doubt as an example. Self-doubt is being uncertain of your capacity to do something right. It's a projection of your own skills into the future, followed by the assumption that your skills might not be sufficient to accomplish the task that you're supposed to do. But who is making these assumptions? Who is deciding that there might be a problem when skills and challenge meet? Your own mind, and nothing or nobody else! And how are you going to oppose yourself?

Again, it's not a problem to consider negative outcomes for a bit; that allows you to try and avoid them. But it's a problem if your mind chooses a negative outcome from the hundreds of different scenarios and sticks with it.

Let's say you have a very difficult pneumonectomy scheduled. Sure, maybe it will be a struggle, but it's also possible that you'll do just fine. Maybe your performance will even be excellent, and you'll surprise everybody, including yourself!

Maybe all surgery will be canceled because the OR gets flooded. (It's not so farfetched; this really happened in New York

78

City during hurricane Sandy.) Who knows, tomorrow morning you might even find a gigantic smoky meteorite crater where the your hospital used to be. Do you see how silly all this is? There are countless possibilities – some more valid than others – but what does the self-doubting mind do? It just sticks to the one scenario where your skills don't match the challenge, sending out a single message: time to worry.

The way you handle external challenges reflects how well you're handling internal challenges. States like self-doubt, fear, uncertainty, and anxiety have a profound effect on our bodies and minds. When we're ridden with self-doubt, our muscles tighten and our heart sinks, leading to a physical and emotional state that sets us up for failure. This way, the negative bias of chatterbox FM easily turns into a self-fulfilling prophecy.

In contrast to external challenges, which you should meet with resolve in order to overcome them and grow from the experience, you can only deal with internal challenges by ignoring them. You cannot beat, outsmart or argue with your own mind. Your mind is a horse that cannot be tamed. In fact, your mind enjoys you trying to tame and control it, because it loves action! Your mind is a player and the more you fight it, the more you're playing along with its game. This fight is completely unfair, because you cannot use your mind to tame your mind. Engaging it is only adding fuel to the fire.

It took me a long time to figure this out. The only way to win the internal challenge is to not accept it in the first place. Do you know what a gauntlet is? A gauntlet is a protective glove that was worn by knights in medieval times. In those days, one knight could challenge another to a duel by throwing one of his gauntlets on the ground. However, the opponent had to pick up the gauntlet to truly accept the challenge. If he didn't, no duel would ensue.

For external challenges, by all means, pick up the gauntlet. Have the world challenge you and become a better person. It's only by checking off accomplished challenges that we can grow and improve ourselves. However, when it comes to the challenge that your own mind throws before you, don't accept. Don't touch the gauntlet.

You might wonder how you can refuse the challenge put forward by your own mind. After all, you can't just walk away from your own head. This is true, but once your inner dialogue takes a negative turn it's possible to just tune it out. This isn't easy, but it can be done if you do two things:

First of all, you need to be aware of the problem. Every time doom and gloom pop up in your mind's eye and every time you get overwhelmed by self-doubt, just recognize it as your mind toying with you. You don't have to immediately fix the problem, but you do need to see the problem.

Secondly, turn off chatterbox FM. Don't listen. Every time a fearful thought pops up, say "Hmm, that's interesting," and move on. Don't dwell on negative thoughts. If the thought dissolves immediately, that's fine. If it sticks around to bother you another hour, that's fine, too. Just don't accept the challenge of fighting your own thoughts!

Ignoring your inner dialogue requires discipline and training. If you find it really difficult, it's probably best to start small. Just ignore your inner ramblings for a few minutes on a given day, and then slowly build it up from there.

Learn to Run Towards Danger

Firefighters are heroes. They're tough. They ride enormous red trucks and they carry heavy equipment with ease. They climb tall ladders that make most of us feel dizzy even by looking at them. But what's even more striking about them is that through training and practice, they've rewired primeval relays deep down in their sympathetic nervous system. When confronted with burning houses, sirens and screaming people, everybody – yes, fire fighters, too – will have a general discharge of the sympathetic nervous system, priming the body to flight or fight. Adrenaline is released in to the bloodstream, aligning the body's functions in order to be able to run as fast as possible. It's a process that's so basic that it's almost impossible to overcome.

And yet while everyone is trying to get out as fast as possible, fire fighters run *into* burning houses. They have learned to run towards danger.

Sometimes as doctors we need to run towards danger, in the sense that we need to consciously take the more difficult path.

One can organize, plan, practice, prepare, and take all possible safety measures, yet problems will occur. Some bad things will hit us even if we did everything to avoid them. This is especially true for surgeries not turning out the way they're expected to. During my residency I quickly noticed that in the management of surgical complications, technical skills represent just one side of the picture. How and when you communicate afterwards is equally important.

I once operated on a young girl who was hit by a golf club. She was standing behind her nephew when he swung the club and the thing hit her left eye with an enormous force.

When she was on the operating table it became clear that the eye was so severely damaged that there was nothing I could to do to save it. She had lost the sight of her left eye forever. I remember that after the surgery one of the first things that popped into my mind was a mental blueprint of our hospital and an estimation where the parents of the young girl could be. The blueprint showed different escape routes that I could take to leave the hospital and avoid meeting the parents. The thought of having to confront them and tell them the bad news made my heart go crazy. But I also knew that if I wasn't going to deliver the painful reality, they would be left in uncertainty. Sooner or later they were going to learn the truth from someone. So I tried to get my act together, and I decided that telling the parents was *my* responsibility and no one else's. When I walked to the nursing ward my heart was pounding. My hands were clammy and the only thing I wanted was to take a 180-degree turn and walk in the other direction. It was as if a giant magnet were pulling me backwards.

But today, what stays in my heart is the memory of the girl's parents thanking me for coming to see them and telling them the bad news in person. They, their son, and their daughter were the ones who had to bear the burden and overcome this terrible accident; treating them with compassion and respect was the least I could do.

When unpleasant things occur, more often that not they're still in your space. While the event itself can't be changed, the communication about it can. The thing to remember is that your space is time dependent. One minute things can be in your reach, and a moment later out of reach. The longer you wait, the more likely it is that solutions will drift away. And once your window of opportunity has passed, problems get a life of their own. It's funny that when you confront your problems head on; quite often you're able to do a significant amount of damage control. On the other hand, procrastination is failure's best friend. If you leave your problems unattended, like weeds in your garden they'll grow.

Face your setbacks head on. Though your orthosympathetic nervous system is trying to make you run away, you need to learn to run towards danger. Problems are like kitchen fires. At first they might be extinguished with a simple glass of water. But if you deny them you'll need a bucket. Or a fire extinguisher. And if you still try to keep them out of your visual field, soon the firefighters will enter your house while you're running out.

Thank God for firefighters – but it's much better to see the first wisps of smoke, respond quickly, and put out your own fire.

4. INTERPERSONAL PERFORMANCE

—m—

Learn to Communicate

People are communicative beings. People like action and interaction. And that's a good thing too, because communication is the oil that makes the cogs in the operating room turn. Without communication, an operating room can't work.

As a surgeon in the OR, there are different categories of people with whom you communicate: your team, the patient, visitors, and sources outside the OR (via intercoms, telephones, pagers); and every category demands its own communication style. However, it goes without saying that your communication with the rest of the team is most important regarding the prevention of mistakes and the enhancement of everybody's performance.

Everybody has a certain communication style, and to a certain extent that's good. We would live in an extremely boring world if everybody had the same style of communication. However, this is not to say that every communication style is efficient and desirable. Some people have obnoxious communication styles, while others seem to be born communicators.

First of all, let me tell you what communication is *not*:

Communication is not something you can misuse without consequences. Everybody has ups and downs, but in the OR it's not a good idea to let everybody know how you're feeling.

It's not just content, but style. Communication needs to be constant for you to be perceived as trustworthy and reliable, but remember that *you will be judged by your worst communication moments*. If your communication style changes with your mood, people will remember you only as a grumpy and bad-tempered person. It doesn't matter if you have you joyful moments in the late afternoon when your early morning mood has vanished. It's the bad communication that sticks.

Communication is not you carrying out a monologue. Bringing your ideas and opinions across when you communicate is just one part of what you should be trying to when you're communicating. If you really want your ideas to reach the other person, you want her to process the information by reflecting on it. Communication means interaction, which in turn means you will not only have to speak but you will also have to listen. For most of us, speaking is the easy part; genuinely listening to what others have to say is a lot more difficult. Only if others reflect upon what you have said and have a chance to comment on that are you one hundred percent sure that the message touched base.

Speech that's aggressive, offensive, or insulting is by no means something that could be labeled as communication. Cursing could be labeled as an *expression* of a frustrated inner state, but *communication* it is not. The same goes for yelling, ranting, and raving. Again, the goal of communication is to get a message across. A message that sticks. If people are offended or frightened, what do they do? They try to forget about the event as soon as possible. And with that they try to forget what was being said.

Oh, and for the sake of completeness, throwing a surgical instrument is not an efficient way of communication either.

When you communicate, first and foremost let respect shine through. Use friendly language and show interest when people respond to you. Avoid looking judgemental, even when the reply you got is not what you expected or what you hoped for. Yes, sometimes people will tell you something that you already know or something that's irrelevant. But what's wrong with replying "thank you" and moving on?

Use clear and precise language. Sloppy communication is among the most important causes of operating room errors, and the reason is that some people use a language that's open to various interpretations. It's unclear communication that leads people to draw their own conclusions and make their own assumptions. If the information that you share with the rest of your team is incomplete, then effectively those who are on the receiving end won't be able to work with a full set of tools.

Also, when you talk to people, make sure you talk singlemindedly. If possible, look them in the eyes and talk directly to them. It's just very difficult to communicate and do something else at the same time. If I'm looking through the microscope, people understand that I cannot take my eyes away from the microscope, so they accept that I talk to them while looking somewhere else. However, if I'm talking and at the same time texting on my cell or writing in the patient's chart, how does that come across? Definitely not as me telling them something that's worth remembering for more than two seconds.

Create a Productive Atmosphere

It can be seducing to focus on small talk. I remember that after ending my fellowship, I came into the hospital one morning and realized I had become a member of staff. Nobody was there to guide me through each and every process, and my task was now to run the show. For some reason, I thought that also involved being an entertainer. To create a congenial atmosphere, I started talking and interacting with everybody around me.

I was wrong. There's no need to give one-man shows in the OR. If you don't like to chat a lot while doing your work, don't feel like you have to. Some of us can talk all day and stay connected to everything that's going on in the OR, while others needs a bit more contemplative focus. Both are perfectly fine, so there's no reason to pretend to be someone you're not. Don't let the fear of silence keep you from doing your job well.

Another way people try to create a pleasant and productive atmosphere is by having music play in the OR. This is a controversial matter, and while some hospitals gladly allow a surgeon to turn on the latest album by Bruce Springsteen before initiating a procedure, it's frowned upon in others. Sure, music can be relaxing. We all enjoy the sensation of gently stirring our laparascopes in patients' bellies while humming along to the sweet voice of Joss Stone. But music can be distracting, too, and might make it hard for some to pay proper attention to their work. Another problem is that tastes vary, and your Verdi-loving colleague may not share your enthusiasm for 1990s grunge music, which can negatively affect his performance if he's made to work while listening to a *Foo Fighters* album.

Personally, I think music in the OR is a good thing, as it keeps people from feeling the need to break silence with mindless chatter. Such chatter is not only much more distracting than music, but can also be a bit tiring. I'd prefer Solomon Burke's deep voice over idle small talk any day! Still, you should never expect music to create a good atmosphere.

In the end, the proper atmosphere is one that's conducive to good, focused work. While you should never feel like you have to entertain the others in the OR, you have some responsibility for creating a positive working environment. However, this is less about cracking jokes and building playlists than it's about making sure that the workload is acceptable, that people treat each other with respect, and that there is trust among everyone involved. Such an atmosphere cannot be built in a day, but requires consistent, careful cultivation. To build trust and respect in the microcosm that is your OR, just treat others with trust and respect. Words carry way less weight than actions – so don't worry about whether you're saying enough to build a good atmosphere, but make sure you're doing enough to make a good atmosphere grow and flourish.

Learn to Read Body Language

Decreasing verbal communication also opens your mind to reading non-verbal communication. Few things make the importance of body language in the OR clearer than robot-assisted surgery, where the surgeon sits in a separate console, stares at a screen, and uses joysticks to manipulate the movements of robotic arms. The usual picture of surgeons standing around the patient dramatically changes here: instead, there are scrub nurses next to the patient and the robot, making sure the robot is positioned correctly while the surgeon sits at a distance.

My brother, who uses a robot to do urology interventions, told me that "the fact that you're separated from the rest of the team is a big disadvantage. When everybody is standing around the operating table, you can look each other in the eyes. It's only now that I can't do that anymore that I realize how much we communicate with our eyes and our body language."

Indeed, even when people's faces are covered by surgical masks, their eyes still provide a wealth of information. A single frown on the scrub nurse's face can tell you something is wrong. The anesthesiologist's big eyes show either that she's impressed or doesn't believe what she's seeing. The resident's sweaty hands betray his stress. There are hundreds of clues like this, informing you of how well (or how badly) things are going. The unspoken truth about what people feel or think can often only be read from their body language.

And so, a good surgeon can read body language. Signs may be subtle and, obviously, reading body language is not an exact science. But that doesn't matter – all these signs have to do is prompt you to ask whether things are going well, or to reassure that sweaty resident that he's doing fine. Body language is an important part of overall communication and should come naturally to most once they start paying attention.

This is what a thoracic surgeon had to say about body language:

"I always thought that there is something magic about body language. That some people were good at reading body language in the OR and I was not. However, I came to see that communication through body language is something that is in fact very natural. It's a skill that everybody possesses. The only thing you have to learn is to open up, to take the leap, and trust your gut feeling. Most bodily signs are so discreet that you cannot put them into words. When I started to pay attention to people's body language in my OR, it changed things dramatically. I felt like I was handed the secret key to a new, much more efficient way of communication. We all have it in us! What do we do in the outpatient clinic? Isn't the communication with our patients based on body language as well? The trick is to be receptive for the signs the person you are talking to is sending."

The flip side to body language is that it's not only about you reading other person's body language. You should also spend some time thinking about the signals you're sending. For example, over the last few years I've noticed that I should watch out for crossing my arms while talking to people. Crossed arms create a distance and a mental wall. It may not be my intention but it looks like a defensive attitude. That's something I don't really want to convey.

So it might be a good idea to replace the crossed arms with a smile. Without wanting to sound too soft, there is nothing that can work miracles like a smile can. Don't ever think that your mask covers the expression of your face. Your eyes will tell.

Don't Push; Make Way

One day one of the junior surgeons entered the small room we called "the aquarium." It was at the end of the corridor that led to the operating rooms, and had large windows all around that enabled one to overview the corridor, the room where patients were prepared for surgery, and the recovery. Because all surgeons came to sit there to write their reports it was the number one place to have a quick chat with your colleagues.

"How do you do that?" she asked me. "You do two cases of surgery while I do one. I'm trying to operate more rapidly but it doesn't feel comfortable. I feel like it's dangerous to try to work so fast."

"Well, don't try to rush your surgery," I said. "Never do that. The secret isn't my surgery. I'm beyond my learning curve now. When I was a junior consultant it took me about two years do reach the optimal balance between speed and safety. After a few years I noticed that trying to increase my speed further would only be dangerous. My complication rate is way below average and I would like to keep it that way, you know. For my patient's sake and especially for my own peace of mind."

She laughed. "Yes, I can see that, but what's the key?"

"I discovered one rule," I said. "Don't push; make way. If you reach the point where you cannot increase your own workflow any more, start to help others to improve theirs. But do it gently. You will have to learn to make way and facilitate. "

People don't like to be pushed. Sure enough, if you push people on the back they'll run a bit faster. If you run after people and yell instructions at them and give them pushes on their back, it may seem that they run faster. However, this is an illusion. What people eventually do is dig their heels into the sand. (Ask yourself – what would *you* do?) Eventually people go slower and slower to compensate for the pushes on their back that they know are going to come.

I know one surgeon that not only verbally tries to make his assistants operate faster, but also begins to physically push their elbows if he thinks that things are not going fast enough.

Have you ever tried to do surgery when someone is pushing your elbow?

Talk about the worst idea ever!

People don't like to be pushed up against the wall either. As a surgeon you have a certain power over people. After all, the captain of a ship not only determines the heading of the ship but also how the ship is run. Up to a certain point, an OR needs a leader, someone who can direct with a firm hand how things go. The fact that for a large part you, the surgeon, have the end responsibility indeed entails that you must (and may) direct people. However, that doesn't mean that you can push people up against the wall. If you dictate to everyone from the morning until the evening what he or she must do, how fast and in what way, it will backfire.

Don't push; make way. What keeps amazing me after all these years is the enormous gain in time and smoothness that you can achieve if you make way for people instead of pushing them. If a subordinate is standing in front of a closed door and you tell this person to walk through the door, they'll turn the doorknob, open the door, and walk through, with the feeling they're doing something that their boss has made them do. However, if you open the door yourself and smile for just a moment, they'll spontaneously walk through the door. Without you even having to say one word – without instruction, without assignment, without pushing! People usually spontaneously choose the easiest and most obvious path. If a door is held open they will step through it.

In my view, instead of instructing people, it's better to look at how you can facilitate. If you yourself pull the sterile sheet across the table, the nurse perhaps can put the instruments on it more quickly. If you help position the patient, the anesthetist meanwhile can check the chart of the patient. If you assemble the laparoscope yourself, in the meanwhile the assistant can cover up the patient. The best thing you can do to get the OR smoothly running is to be constantly in "scanning mode" for opportunities to pitch in.

For many little actions, it's true that it's faster to do it yourself instead of instructing someone to do it!

Look around for the small things you can do to improve the flow of activity. And not only for the aspect of time – the saving of time is just a beneficial side effect. It's about showing involvement. If you do your best to let other people execute their jobs more smoothly, then that will be greatly appreciated. People will notice and they'll surely appreciate you for it. And you'll be in the aquarium writing your report that much sooner.

Be Consistent

We all know fickle surgeons. The only constant in their lives is their unpredictability. Most of us have a few in our immediate surroundings: they can be extremely nice one day and outright hostile the next. They can praise the skills of their scrub nurse on Monday and chastise her for some minor issue on Tuesday. I've come across many of them myself.

One day, I plucked up my courage and asked one of them about their behavior. "Miriam," I said, "you're a bit of a capricious person. You can be amiable one minute, and crabby the next. Sometimes, you seem to be overly passionate about your work, and other times you seem not to care at all. This does not seem to be related to stress or the time of day. It's completely random. I wonder, are you unaware of your inconsistency, or is it behavior that you're perfectly conscious of?"

"Of course I am conscious of it!" she said. "Being capricious is what brings me respect. People are intrigued by the fact that what I do or say cannot be predicted, and that leads to a certain admiration. I enjoy it! If I enter the room, I keep people on the edges of their seats! People stay on edge because they don't know what I'm about. Everybody works a bit better because of it."

If only she knew what people really thought when she entered the room... it certainly wasn't about respect. Every tirade decreases workplace respect. Sure, being inconsistent puts people on edge. But that doesn't make them more productive. On the contrary, people need to know what they can expect from you. Being consistent does not only provide your colleagues with much-needed grip; it's a necessary condition for collaboration, just like honesty, impeccability, reliability and integrity. Those characteristics are more than something that is simply NTH (nice to have). They are the cornerstones of good and long-lasting teamwork.

Consistency breeds confidence. If people know with whom they're dealing, they feel safe and won't fear being taken by surprise. In the end, trust is related to our expectancies of the future: are the reactions and actions of people around us predictable? If so, we feel that "things will turn out all right." Consistency builds relationships. As people feel good around others who are consistent, these others become social magnets, attracting people to their surroundings.

The opposite is also true: fickle people will get into conflicts with everyone around them, thereby creating a social vacuum that is actively avoided by others.

Miriam, the colleague mentioned above, experienced exactly that. People made a special effort not to be scheduled together with her! Nurses and residents struck deals (mostly involving chocolate cake) to minimize their exposure to Miriam.

And, perhaps more significantly, if your colleagues and assistants don't respect you, they won't go the extra mile to save you when you make a mistake. Your consistent and respectful treatment of them creates a reservoir of good will that can help you when you really need it.

Consistency saves energy, too. If you know what to expect, you'll be at ease. Steady people are mental energy preservers. The less cognitive resources your team spends on guessing your mood, the more they have left to focus on their jobs. There is nothing more tiring to people than having to anticipate every possible scenario when they deal with other people.

Now, consistency does not mean being boring. Don't be afraid of people thinking you lack personality or spine just because you try to maintain a predictable character. You can be whoever you want to be and you can express style, dynamics, innovation, one-liners, and 1970s hairdo's to your liking. Go for it, but know what you stand for and stick to it!

Staying consistent can be hard, though. If you insist on having everybody in the OR at 7:50 AM sharp, you cannot arrive at 8:15 AM yourself, just because your newborn kept you up all night. Consistency does not mean *most of the time*. It does not mean *when life is easy*. It means *always*.

Don't Blame

One of my friends told me the story of when he was a resident. Scrubbing in with the surgeon, Dr. Jones, was fun. That is to say, if you could see the irony of things. Jones was a tall, good-looking guy of about fifty. He wore dark horn-rimmed glasses that gave him a stern face. Together with his sturdy build this contributed to a certain appearance that represented a negative personality. He always told his residents that he would not only teach them orthopedics, he would also give them lessons in what he called sociology, meaning long tirades about how screwed up the health care system was. He could rant on for hours about the fact that he disliked being a surgeon, that he could have more money if he had not made the mistake of studying medicine.

Now one day Dr. Jones was in the OR doing a small bone graft to fix an ankle problem. It was not an easy operation. A small piece of bone had to be carved out of the hip bone and shaped meticulously to fit exactly in the ankle joint. My friend was just doing the first weeks of his residency and was not invited to scrub in. He was just standing in the corner of the OR as an observer of this long and difficult surgery.

As the hours passed, it became more and more difficult to stay awake. As he was standing there, he didn't realize that he had crossed his arms and was silently tapping on this left upper arm with his right index finger.

Jones suddenly turned red, straightened his back and started to call him all sorts of names. He screamed, "Who the hell do you think you are? I can see that extremely annoying tapping of your finger out

100

of the corner of my eye. Do you have any idea how distracting that is? This surgery stinks and it's all your fault!" As everybody froze in the OR he faced the operating field again and muttered to himself, "Finally I'll be able to concentrate. How does a guy have to work here?"

Now isn't that strange? I mean this surgeon was six foot five inches tall and yet had a personality so small it could fit in the palm of your hand.

Often when people come to address human performance, they begin from the standpoint of errors, mistakes and disasters. They analyze what isn't working or hasn't worked so that they can "fix" the problem. This approach, however, immediately puts them at a psychological disadvantage, because of course instead of thinking positive, inspiring thoughts that will motivate them to improve, they're focusing on depressing, negative ones.

That's not to say that preventing errors isn't important, because of course it is. But tackling the issue from a negative viewpoint only creates a blame culture in which the "culprit" is named and shamed, and leads to an investigation into what could have been done to prevent the situation from arising in the first place.

If things blow up in our faces, more often than not there is one person who is to blame. One person did something stupid. One person made a mistake. So what is the quick-fix route to improving human performance? We're going to kindly ask this person not to do that anymore, and we're going to explain to the rest of the team that they are not supposed to act in the way this person did. Problem solved. And dealing with the initial human mistake is easy because it's tangible. You can pinpoint the wrongdoer. You can pinpoint the culprit. You can pinpoint the bad apple.

For example, take wrong site surgery. In this case, there is clearly one person to blame: the surgeon holding the knife. He performed poorly and should make sure to take better care in the future. So show him the error of his ways and use his case to illustrate why everybody should always focus.

Something about this scenario seems too simple, too pat.

Let's think about this. If a surgeon was able to initiate a wrong site surgery, there must also be something wrong at the level of interpersonal performance, since apparently nobody else noticed the mistake, or at least nobody spoke up. Things may also not be okay at the organizational level: was there a checklist or a protocol installed? If so, why didn't it work?

So yes, the surgeon made the mistake. However, blaming only him is too easy, because his team and the organization also let him down. Human mistakes only lead to disasters if the microcosm as a whole isn't functioning well, and if there aren't enough checks and balances in place. While *someone* should have done things differently, blaming this *someone* isn't going to help anybody. The culture of blame only leads to a situation in which everybody tries not to be the person making the next mistake. What you instead want is an environment in which people also watch out for the mistakes of others.

To get to such an environment, it's important to let go of the blame game and to focus on learning from mistakes. Instead of seeing failures as negative elements, they should be seen as stepping stones. It's counterintuitive to think positively about mistakes, but really, they allow us to grow and improve – personally, as a team and as an organization.

Lead by Example

How can you and your team meet all the challenges mentioned here? How can you make sure that everybody stays focused, that people come in well prepared, that the work atmosphere breeds performance, that mistakes are collectively avoided, and that surgery in the OR reaches optimal flow?

For any microcosm, regardless of whether it is an OR, a submarine, or an airplane's cockpit, you can ask whether a leader is needed. Does the ship need a captain charting the course? Is there a need for one person who makes sure that the whole team is following the same path?

To me, the answer is definitely "yes." There's no doubt in my mind: if you want your microcosm to move somewhere, if you want everybody to be on the same page, you definitely need leadership.

If you remove leadership even a well-organized system will rapidly fall apart, because leadership brings together people working in demanding environments. It's part of the structure of the microcosm and offers guidance. Also, a strong leader makes people feel safe and confident.

To me, the most important reason why people perform better when guided by a strong leader is that they can take their minds off the bigger picture. If people are convinced that they are being led towards the right destination, they have more time and energy to spend on the here-and-now of things. There's also less energy spent on discussing where to go, because the leader makes that high-level decision.

This is not the same as blind obedience. I am not saying that there's one person telling the rest what to do. Even if he'd want to, people these days won't accept authority like that! The days of top-down management are over, and rest assured, they will never come back.

Encouraging people to think for themselves and giving them some part in decision-making only improves performance. If you're the surgeon in charge in the operating room, you'd better have a crew around you that dares to speak up when you're about to make a mistake. (Do you think anyone on Miriam's crew would dare speak up? Hardly!) This means being an approachable leader and not insisting on absolute authority.

Of course, a fine balance is necessary to make this work. If every choice becomes a collective decision, you lose part of the benefits of leadership. If no one has any say, the microcosm is as good as your performance. What you need to do is value and consult people's opinions, while keeping the final say. Make sure you use everyone in the OR as a safety net for your actions, but also ensure they trust your judgment and leadership. If you strike the right balance, you can create a microcosm in which all obstacles to high performance can be overcome.

To put it simply, follow these guidelines:

1. If it's a simple and obvious question, make the decision yourself.

2. If you want to provide instruction, ask for opinions, then make your decision. Do not criticize the opinions; simply explain why you made your choice.

3. If you want input, ask for opinions, then make your decision.

4. If you cannot decide, find someone with more experience and consult. Then make your decision.

You can see that every option ends the same way: "make your decision." The differences are in the process.

For those who doubt whether the input of others can be valuable to a surgeon, I have the following anecdote, which was told to me by a very experienced surgeon.

"I've been doing surgery for a long time and I always thought that there was just one person responsible for everything going on in the OR. Since I knew best, I was telling others what to do. I got so used to depending on my own opinion that I didn't even consider the opinions of others. What could a surgeon with twenty years of experience learn from a resident or a nurse?

"Then one day, I was doing cataract surgery and I was about to implant the intraocular lens, when all of a sudden a first year resident – a real newbie – asked me to reconsider the implant I was going to use. Having looked at the calculations himself, he thought it was the wrong one. My first reaction was a mix of disbelief and anger. Why, he's got some nerve to doubt me! I had just checked the lens calculations myself. Anyway, since the whole OR was looking in my direction, I thought it would be a good idea to quickly review the readings and the lens calculations, just to nip in the bud this outburst of disbelief.

"Surely enough, I had the wrong lens in my hand! Instead of implanting a lens with a power of sixteen diopters, I was mistakenly planning to implant one of twenty-six diopters. Almost double, and completely wrong! Now that was a good lesson in humility. So you see, you'd better be nice to everyone around you, even to the rookies. You never know who's going to save the day."

You Need a Mentor

Three millimeters. How long is three millimeters? About the length of an ant? The width of a knitting needle? The battery logo on top of your iPhone? The head of a match?

Three millimetres was the width of the point of the blade that I had in my hands to put the knife into an eye for the first time of my life. Actually it's nearly nothing, three millimeters You have to look closely to be able to see it. And yet for an eye, the blade of a knife of three millimeters is gigantic. The smallest wrong movement can cause a bleed or a scar. The difference between seeing and not seeing. It was October 2000. The Rotterdam Eye Hospital. One of the biggest and most renowned eye hospitals in the world. And in one of the six operating rooms of this big institute, there was a small resident. With a knife of three millimeters in his right hand and drops of sweat between his shoulder blades. While I looked through the microscope into the eye of the patient, I asked myself, "Actually the question is… who ever had the nerve to think of this? Where do you get the courage to be the first to put a knife in to – according to me – the most precious and most beautiful organ of the human body?"

Yes, I had prepared everything to the smallest detail. I had practiced hours in the lab: Sitting still and looking trough the oculars of the microscope. Learning to control the slightest movements of my hands. Learning tying knots under the microscope, knots that are too small to see with the naked eye. I had studied everything in textbooks. I had been sitting next to my supervisors in the operating room while I assisted them. I had memorized every movement as well as I could and then when the OR session was over I had noted everything carefully in my big notebook.

And yet preparation isn't everything. Just like a relay runner passes the stick to the next runner, preparation must become confidence. And that's where it hurts when you have to do something for the first time. After all, confidence is a tower of blocks. Each little success is a new block. You can build further on each new accomplishment. But what if there is not a single block yet? What if it's something that you have never done before in real life? Yes, you can prepare, but how can you be one hundred percent sure that something will work if your track record *for real* is zero?

While I brought the blade closer and closer to the eye my heart began to beat harder and harder. The lenses of my glasses became steamy because of my face getting red. My hands. My God, my hands. The hands that I could hold so perfectly still during my practice sessions were shaking. Tremor! The biggest taboo of any surgeon. The sign of weakness, stress, tension, incertitude! (That's what I thought back then; now I know better. In the OR, there is room for shaky hands if you know how to deal with it.)

It got worse. Around the eye there was some sort of force field that made it impossible for me to bring the blade closer! It seemed as if an invisible rubber protective coating was surrounding the eye that I couldn't penetrate. I couldn't bring myself to bring the blade closer to the eye.

I felt like a parachutist seated on the edge of the opened door of the plane, ready for his first jump, wrapped in the deafening sound of the roaring engines and the wind. That split second before the leap when your visual field is so narrow that you feel like you're looking through a gun barrel.

What in God's sake makes you jump? Well, that's pretty simple. Your mentor. Your instructor. Your trainer. He or she says to you, "Come on, you can do it!" and gives you a little push in the back if needed.

I can assure you I have been *very* lucky with my mentors. The time and energy that was spent on training me and making me the surgeon I am today is just beyond imagination. On a professional level, the training I got from my mentors was the greatest gift I could ever receive. However this is not to say that I got things for free. In life, there is no thing such as a free ride. I think this is where a lot of interns, residents, and fellows get it wrong. Those who think that good mentoring is like a gift that's randomly thrown around should have a closer look. There is very little luck involved, and definitely very little arbitrariness. If you want a mentor to guide you, rest assured you will have to earn it. And no, I don't mean it can be bought with money, ice cream, or short skirts. I am sorry.

From my experience, the relationship between a mentor and a pupil is a two way street. Giving and taking from *both* parties is required. Indeed, *both* parties have something to bring to the table. First, what's in it for the pupil? Of course, the knowledge, the training, the schooling. Learning. Being guided while taking the first steps into unfamiliar territory. That's all easily understood. But what is often overlooked is the fact that there is also something in it for the mentor, and that's the pleasure of the passed on knowledge. To a mentor it's not really the passing on itself that's valuable. At least I don't know any mentors that genuinely like to talk someone else through their job while they would do it better, more safely, and faster themselves. That's no fun. It's the moment when the knowledge hits home, when it resonates in the pupil, when they see their knowledge being used by others. That's fulfilling.

It's taboo to discuss it openly, but we all know that not every student, every resident, every intern, or every fellow gets the same training. On paper they do. In real time they don't.

Phew. I'm glad we got that over with. Did I really say that? Yes I did. I'll do it again. *Not everybody gets the same training*. Good mentors are hard to come by and if you want good mentoring, you'll have to earn it. I know there are national guidelines for the kind and number of surgeries that residents ought to do. But that doesn't change the reality that it's very hard to claim real mentorship.

Yes, to residents who want everything to be handed to them on a silver platter this will sound as a downright bummer. For the I-wanna-have-what-they're-having it's an unfair system, it's against the hospital's policy, and it's a shame. But hey, don't shoot the messenger. I didn't design this planet! This is how the game of mentoring works. You can't win the game without playing along.

The good news is that you can choose to be different, you can choose to earn what you think you should have. If you're prepared to walk the extra mile, you'll reap the benefits tenfold! And while your colleagues are moaning about the fact that it's a disgrace that they weren't allowed to scrub in on that coronary bypass, you'll be *doing* the coronary bypass!

As the saying goes, there are no traffic jams on the extra mile. Many are called, but few are chosen. That's why it's easy to walk the extra mile. The only thing you need to do is to make sure you have the right attitude and that you're willing to put in the work.

5. ORGANIZATIONAL PERFORMANCE

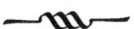

Start the Habit of Ticking Off

There is one simple action that can improve the quality of surgical care more than any new surgical technique, any new piece of equipment, or any new instrument. It's something that can be implemented all over the world, in any hospital, in any city, and in any field of surgery. It will save more lives than any procedure you or I can ever think of. It's something that we can learn from other fields of high performance, like aviation and oil drilling.

It's the use of checklists.

Checklists are going to save the day.

I'll tell you a story of something that happened to me a long time ago. I was in the operating room, preparing for the next case. The next operation on the list was a cataract operation that was planned to be performed under retrobulbar local anesthesia. For this kind of anesthesia we use a mixture of scandicaine and mepivacaine in ophthalmology – both potent local anesthetics – and inject them with a long needle behind the eye. This anesthetizes the eyeball, paralyses the muscles of the eye, and makes the eye blind for a couple of hours because it shuts down the optic nerve. Although the effect of the injection wears off after a couple of hours, it's not a trivial little prick.

I was looking at the patient's chart. The pre-op plan had already been filled in; it was the right eye that had to be operated.

Suddenly I heard a noise behind me, looked over my shoulder, and a saw a bald, friendly old man in the operating chair. He was looking in my direction. Apparently one of the nurses had brought the man to the operating room, put him in the chair, and had left the OR without saying a word. Whereas one minute before I was alone in the OR, now this gentle man had joined me.

I decided to get on with things. I looked at the chart and asked, "Are you Mr. Vanden Bergh?"

"Yes," the man said with a soft grating voice.

"Is your birthday 8 December 1923?" I asked.

"Yes," he said again, still smiling at me. I grabbed the syringe with the anesthetic and walked towards him.

When I came closer, he opened his mouth and closed his eyes. I stopped. This was just not what people do when they're going to get an injection behind the eye. Normally they open their eyes widely and look straight at me. And they certainly don't open their mouth!

I took the chart and asked the patient what his name was.

"Yes," was the answer.

I came a bit closer and asked him again "What's your name?"

Again "yes" was the answer. And despite I had the feeling that there was something completely wrong with this picture, the man kept smiling at me. So I leaned forward. "Sir! What's your name?"

"Oh, my name? Jansen!" he said.

Shivers ran down my spine.

What seemed to be the case? This nice man was stone deaf. He was – as is often the case with people with hearing loss – ashamed that he couldn't understand a word of what was being said to him. He didn't want to be a burden to anyone so he answered everything with a "yes" and a smile.

The mindblowing thing was that this man who was sitting in the operating chair in the ophthalmology operating room didn't even need an eye operation. He had come to the hospital for a dental prosthesis! Because the stomato ward was overcrowded he was transferred to the ophthalmology ward. Every single person that contributed to his transfer from the ward to the OR had asked closed questions (questions to be answered with a "yes" or a "no").

Are you Mr. Vanden Bergh? "Yes!"

Are you here for cataract surgery? "Yes!"

Is your surgery scheduled at ten o'clock? "Yes!"

Would an appointment for a postop visit tomorrow at three in the afternoon be fine? "Yes!"

And so on. No wonder he opened his mouth when I approached him, pointing a shiny needle in the direction of his face. He was here for a dental prosthesis, and I thought I was looking at the perfect candidate for cataract surgery.

Would a checklist have prevented this near-catastrophe? The answer is yes. Going over a simple checklist, asking *open* questions ("What's your name? What's your birthday? What's the intervention you're coming for?") would have nipped this error in the bud very early. This patient would never even have left the nursery ward. And for me, I would never have asked closed questions if I knew back then how this can get you in trouble.

I would have gathered the *whole team* in the OR (the anesthesiologist, the resident, the nurse) and we would have checked the patient's name and birthday, the kind of surgery, and the eye that was going to be operated *together* by asking the patient *open questions*. Just as I do now before starting any surgical procedure in Medifocus, my own eye surgery clinic. And I mean *any* surgical procedure, big or small.

Of course checklists are not the answer to all problems. Every new checklist is a new piece of administration you will have to deal with. So checklists ought to used sparingly. I once saw the most intensive form of bureaucracy in the patient's charts of a hospital. They had developed so many checklists that they had to put a checklist on top of the charts to check off filling in all the checklists inside the chart. Checklists of checklists!

Checklists should be:
- Simple and direct.
- As brief as possible.
- To the point.
- Focused on preventing the most serious or most common mistakes.

Checklists should *not* be:

- Open to interpretation.
- About minor issues.
- Complicated and time consuming.
- Optional.

Human knowledge and reliability are limited. Humans make mistakes – sometimes because of a lack of experience, sometimes because of fatigue, and sometimes just because. We face complex mechanisms in the operating room, and quite often the tools we have to do a good job aren't equal to the potential flaws and pitfalls. We just can't just solely rely on experience, intelligence, gut feeling, and teamwork anymore. We need checklists to serve as a background layer of control. We need a mechanism that endorses our thinking and the actions we're about to take. Just like it's impossible for a plane to depart before all topics on the pilot's checklists are checked off, you should start the habit of ticking off also.

Walk the Protocol Minefield

I know of one hospital that treated all employees to cake because there was something to celebrate. In fact, the management announced that this event was huge, a real milestone in the history of the hospital.

The digital system that contained all the hospital's protocols had reached the magical number of one thousand.

I kid you not, a thousand. Yes, a thousand!

What is there to celebrate when an organization buries its people under a thousand protocols? Could somebody please explain how people are actually supposed to deal with a thousand protocols? The problem is that there is an enduring illusion at the organizational level and that's the idea that when it comes to protocols, more is better. More and more protocols are developed every day in a hopeless effort to try to make sure people are doing what they are supposed to do. Unfortunately, there is nobody who is going to have a close look at the protocols that are already there. In most organizations, nobody has the task of deleting unnecessary protocols or combining several protocols into one. So what happens is an unlimited proliferation. To me, this is more dangerous than having no protocols at all.

Imagine six people in an operating room, ready to start a procedure that involves the heart-lung machine. The machine comes with a plastic disposable valve that needs to be connected in a specific way. This manoeuvre is a bit tricky so there is a protocol that describes how to connect the valve.

116

Person A and B know that there's a protocol and know what it's saying. So far so good. Person C and D know there's a protocol but they have never read it. Yet, there is no immediate problem, because they can look it up if need so. Person E and F don't even know that there is a protocol.

Now this is asking for problems. First of all, because if E and F need to handle the valve they might just connect it like they think it's okay. That might mess things up. However, there is a second, less obvious problem, and that is this. Most likely A, B, C and D are going to assume that everybody in the room, including E and F, know the protocol. Most people will feel like everything is covered once there is a protocol in place, and most people will expect everybody to conform. Working with protocols can be the cause of errors because as much as we need protocols in the OR, they also give a false feeling of safety. Working with protocols is a minefield.

Let's be bold and ask, what *is* a protocol? Too often protocols are seen as what they are not. They are seen as easy-fix solutions to problems. As if creating a protocol will make people do what you had in mind as a solution for that particular problem. A protocol is not a guarantee that people are – or aren't – going to do something, it's just a document that is somewhere in the database; no more, no less. Really, it's solely and utterly a document. This document describes the guidelines and agreements that need to be followed. You can draw up a protocol for almost everything. There are protocols describing the guidelines for a diagnostic, how to manage a treatment of some kind of disease, the magical preparation of medicines, or even to explain what equipment you need for what kind of surgery.

As mentioned above, having a protocol in place doesn't necessarily mean that people are doing what the protocol says. A couple of requirements need to be met before people are going to actually do what the protocol says.

- The amount of protocols must be limited. No matter how efficient a digital system can be, when a system counts hundreds of protocols, it can be very hard to find the needed document, and thus having a large number is a disadvantage.

- People need to be trained in how to use the system, whether it's analogue on paper or digital. The system then needs to be used on a regular basis by everyone. This is not always easy. Consider the actual logistics of hundreds of employees accessing a digital protocol database. The amount of passwords someone can remember? Well, I really hope it's at least five, but this is probably way too optimistic. Sure we can give people a login code for a very complex digital system, but since most people are already flooded with logins and passwords, the odds will be very good that after one week they'll lose their specific login name that was dropped in their mailbox and quickly deleted afterwards. And yes, that password... was it the name of the dog added by a reverse date of birth of my youngest son, or was it just 123abc?

- The protocols themselves need to be as simple and clear as possible. Protocols that are long and complicated and have a decision scale that is even longer just depress people. Protocols need to be there on hand when we need them and in our work area where it's very busy!

- Protocols need to be managed from within the hospital. Someone needs to be responsible for this, and not only to make sure that they are up to date but also to modify then and to remove any protocols that are overlapping or duplicated. If not, the protocols within your system will grow like Haemophilus influenzae bacteria on a chocolate agar.

Protocols are, and will be, guidelines. Some are soft and reasonably open, others are tough and require extremely good reasons to try to divert from them. You always need to realize one thing: a protocol is made to describe what you need to do in *most cases*. Not a single protocol is so sophisticated that it gets all exceptions and unforeseen circumstances. The reason for this is that you would not be able to work with a protocol that is one hundred percent complete and covers everything because it would look as incomprehensible as a credit card contract. That's why there are exceptional situations that may arise in which you do not follow protocols. No protocol relieves you from the task of using your brains. You and only you are responsible for your actions, and if you think protocols will make your life easier because you won't need to think for yourself anymore you might be heading for some bare-knuckle lessons on how the world really works. The thing of it is, mind and memory are two different things. The best way to look at protocols is as an extension of your memory. You cannot remember everything and so protocols are there to support your memory. The thinking part, however, is completely up to you, and even a thousand protocols cannot replace common sense and analytical thinking.

Pour Yourself Into It

No matter what kind of profession you do, the only way to stay motivated for life is to put your heart and soul into your job. And if you do, you'll create personalized habits that translate into your individual approach.

Over the course of the years every surgeon develops his or her tricks. Specific things that no one else does. It can be putting some stitches just slightly deeper than your colleague just to make sure that the knob holds better or even the way you hold the needle holder. It can be a form that you have created to make an OR report faster. You just have to cherish traits as they translate who you are.

If you pour yourself in to your work, you will radiate one of the most appreciated characteristics that someone who is working with patients can have: authenticity. Of course, patients want first and foremost someone who is skilled, well trained, and knows both the literature and the practical applications. But there is more to a doctor-patient relationship than technical details and craftsmanship. In my view, patients are equally keen on finding someone who is authentic. Someone who is honest. Someone who stands tall in every situation.

I am convinced that surgeons who do not like their jobs cannot provide good surgery. I mean, not all the time. Look, surgery sometimes feels like a routine. Maybe not during the first couple of years of your career but at some point you might feel like you're standing in front of an assembly line in a factory. That's why if you want to continue loving your job, you need to pour everything you've got into it. That special sewing technique you thought of – why don't you give it a name? And if you think that your trick is much better than what others do, then there's nothing wrong with bragging about it and sharing it with others. It really is the best remedy against a burnout.

To me, one of the best examples is Dr. Claes H. Dolhman. He is a leading eye surgeon at the very well known Massachusetts Eye and Ear Infirmary in Boston, Massachusetts. He's a very friendly man and one of the developers of the Boston Keratoprothesis, an artificial cornea that allows people with a cloudy cornea to regain their sight.

He's well known for having boundless enthusiasm for his innovation. His life's work fills him with enthusiasm, and even after decades of practice his eyes still shine when he talks about how the artificial cornea helps people live better lives. It's wonderful to see the power of associating who you are deep inside with the actions that you undertake.

While most of us don't have an invention that helps the blind to see, we do have our own experiences. Share them with others. Pouring yourself into your work and sharing your knowledge is what keeps the flame burning.

Organize Everything at Your Fingertips

Abraham Lincoln reportedly once said, "If I had sixty minutes to cut down a tree, I would spend forty minutes sharpening the axe and twenty minutes cutting down the tree." Preparation is everything. If you want to reach flow in the observation-action cycle mentioned above, you need to have an environment that's as predictable and familiar as possible. After all, surgery itself comes with enough unpredictability!

Still, there are plenty of surgeons who are more than willing to skip preparation. They have a good lunch, head into the scrub room, wash their hands, put on their gloves and apron, and sit down behind the microscope. Here's what unfolds over time:

13:48 – First incision.

13:50 – "I need a 1.2 sideport knife!"

13:51 – "Do we have an IV?"

13:54 – "Can someone find me the depth adjustable diamond blade?"

14:02 – "Would you call supplies and see if that lens implant I ordered arrived?"

14:15 – "Oh, we're out of blank DVDs. Can someone call the store downtown and have some brought in through FedEx? Tell them it's *urgent*."

14:16 – "Hey... where did everybody go?"

Now, the excuse for this behavior is that surgeons are action-oriented and want to get down to business. This is perfectly understandable. However, hunting down medication, prosthetics, and patient files during surgery takes time. Valuable time.

One minute of preparation can save ten minutes of lost time during surgery. So if you're really about action, make sure you come in prepared!

One of the first things to do before surgery is to check everything you can. Do this before you're wearing sterile clothing! You yourself can get a lot done at this stage, without having to work through others. Run through the most likely scenarios of the surgery. How long will it take? Which instruments are standard? What extras are needed? Do you need donor blood to be available? Prosthetics? Which sutures do you want? Scoop? Cauter?

Divide your toolkit into three categories:

1. Instruments, sutures and prosthetics that you will definitely need. These need to be sterile and available straight away.

2. Instruments you will probably need. Make sure they're available in the OR, within reaching distance. Make sure the circulating nurse knows where they are.

3. Instruments you probably won't need. Make sure everybody knows where they are, in case they are needed anyway.

Brief your whole team before you go into surgery. Discuss what the procedure is about, how long it will take, and what the focus points are. Try to estimate the experience of those around you, including their technical know-how and how well they know their way around the OR.

Before you put on sterile clothing, properly adjust the settings of the equipment as much as you can. Personally, I'm known for preparing every single detail before scrubbing. Before I head into the scrub room I even make sure the cables on the floor, the surgery light, and the mp3 player volume are all exactly as I want them. Doing things yourself is usually a lot quicker than asking someone else to do it for you – I can adjust the speaker volume in three seconds, but if I ask someone else to do it, it always takes them three minutes!

Good preparation leads to good flow and focus, and they in turn lead to quicker surgery with a lower risk of complications and faster patient recovery. What you need is a clear plan of action and your tools at your disposal.

Comments on Live Surgery

Live surgery should be more controversial than it is today. The entertainment value of live surgery is clear, and at any conference it's usually the talk of the day. It appeals to many of our emotions, like tension, insecurity, anxiety, joy... and so you'd think there would also be an emotion-laden debate about it. You would expect live surgery to have its fair share of advocates and detractors.

However, this isn't the case. Live surgery is commonplace at many conferences. In fact, some conferences consist *solely* of live surgery! Now is the lack of controversy due to the safety of live surgery? Is it just as safe as other forms of operating and is no discussion necessary? Is its educational value as much as proponents say it is? Or is it just universally tolerated because it's entertaining?

I don't want to insult anyone by bringing this up. Live surgery is usually done by highly experienced surgeons. Only carefully selected experts are allowed to operate on patients while being broadcast. This should lower the odds of complications – at least theoretically. Also, live surgery is pure surgery. A surgeon cannot edit the video to only show his finest hours; if he gets into trouble while being broadcast, he cannot hide from his mistakes. These mistakes are instructive for the audience, so live surgery does indeed contribute to the spread of medical knowledge.

Still, the lack of discussion on the topic surprises me. In my personal experience, live surgery often involves surgeons struggling with the new equipment, tools, and staff that come with an

OR that they are not familiar with. As I explained earlier, routine can be your best friend if you need to perform, but there is nothing routine about live surgery, especially if it's performed by a guest surgeon in an unfamiliar OR. And even if the surroundings are familiar, the added stress of live surgery does not always translate in increased performance.

Also, the entertainment value sometimes leaves a bad taste in my mouth. Yes, it is *pure* surgery. Mistakes are made. However, if I notice an audience hardly paying attention until these mistakes or complications arise, I get the feeling they have been waiting for drama. Once the bad parts of surgery become highlights, you have to wonder about ethical implications.

Behind the scenes, live surgery can turn ugly. After a complicated surgery and once the video feed had been turned off, I once saw a surgeon throw away his tools. He collected his gear, walked out without saying a word, jumped into his car, and drove away with screeching tires. The lack of self-confidence that follows episodes like these can be an issue for months, or even years.

So while live surgery certainly has its place in the medical community, it makes sense to see if we can get rid of the more negative aspects. If you agree to perform live surgery, you might want to take the following into account:

• Be selective about the cases you accept. Try and stay in full control over the admitted patients and indications. If you're in doubt about performing live surgery for a given case, don't do it.

• Keep your surroundings familiar. You should always prefer your own OR and your own hospital. If that's not possible, because you'll be acting as a guest surgeon, do try and operate using your own tools. The needle holder you know will give you confidence, as will your own scrub nurse. Don't worry about that second plane ticket: the advantage of having someone you know with you in the OR is certainly worth it.

• Try and get a good idea of the whole set-up. Ask how the session will be organized, how many people will be present in the OR, who will be responsible for anesthesia, what equipment will be available, and who will be on stand-by for technical assistance. Only agree to live surgery if you trust the setting enough to operate on a member of your own family in there!

• Visit the OR in advance, in a relaxed manner. Don't do this on the day of the live surgery, as it will be busy with preparations. Try and visit the day before. Boot the equipment and become familiar with the machines, tools, and microscopes.

• Limit the amount of people in the OR as much as possible during live surgery. Technicians and colleagues have a habit of swamping the OR during live surgery, but they will only bring chaos to the room. Be firm and only keep the people who you need in the room. Ask the others to leave.

• Focus on your job during the live surgery, not on the audience. Even if there is a live audio feed, you're there to communicate with your team and not with the viewers. You can talk to them afterwards!

Live surgery does not offer ideal circumstances for high performance in the OR. Even so, you can improve these circumstances and optimize the procedure. By taking time and adding energy and preparation, you can make live surgery sessions safer.

I'm not looking to create a full controversy here. I'm not even looking for a discussion on the balance between advantages and risks of live surgery. I just think we should talk more about the ways in which to improve the practice of live surgery. We can make it safer and more effective and so we should. If live surgery improves, everybody wins. Not in the least bit our patients.

Dealing with Mistakes and Setbacks

No matter what kind of precautions we take, no matter how we good we are, complications will always arise. You know what's said: "A surgeon without complications is a surgeon with a bad memory." Indeed, I might want to add, "A surgeon without complications might also sit on his backside all of the time."

Most complications take us by surprise. Quite often, it's not even the difficult operations in which we're caught by surprise. It's the routine operations, the operations where we assumed the risk was low.

When complications occur, they hit us hard on the inside. Complications are stark confrontations with our own limitation, mistakes, and shortcomings. They're the images that are still burned in our retina when we wake up at night. Complications are troublesome but they are part of life, our life.

Complications and mistakes undermine our self-confidence. After a mishap, the confidence that we need the very next day just slides through our fingers.

No matter how difficult it might be, the only way to deal with complications is to analyze, act and move on.

First of all, analyze. This is difficult – usually, in case of a complication the only thing we want to do is to run away and stop thinking about it. We would rather run the New York marathon three times in a row than to face reality. But sooner or later we'll need to analyze what went wrong, so why don't we find out as soon as possible? Analyze and discover what went wrong, and share that information with others. Because you're so emotionally involved with what went wrong, the best way is to involve others. These can be your working colleagues, the hospital board, or even the medical liability insurer.

The worst possible thing you can do is hide in your office.

Secondly, you must act. Look at it from a distance and ask others' advice. See what can be improved in order to prevent the same thing from happening again. Do you need to gain more knowledge? Is there a need for a checklist? A new protocol? Other agreements? Decide what the best approach would be to prevent it from recurring, and implement this as soon as possible.

And last but not least.... Move on. It is said that our mind always focuses on the negative. This is why the primary function of our mind is to survive, to see dangers. Our mind is easily focused on the negative. Research even shows us that you need five positive experiences to counterweigh one negative, and this is due to the fact that negative experiences carry a lot of weight. That's why it's so easy to get stuck in the past. Negative memories are like quicksand – you just get stuck in them.

Mel Brooks, the famous actor, said, "As long as the world is turning and spinning, we are going to be dizzy and we are going to make mistakes." And it's true enough. As long as people are going to do *anything*, things will go wrong. As long as surgeons are going to get out of bed in the morning, get dressed, and drive to the hospital to help people get better, complications will occur.

The only thing you can do is to minimize the chance of errors occurring and to create a microcosm that is as worry-free as possible. Because in the end, it's the absence of worry that enables people to outperform themselves. It's the freedom from worry that makes people excel. And this freedom comes from knowing that you did everything you could to do your job as well as possible.

Take care of the three layers of performance. At the personal level, make sure you're as prepared as you can be. At the interpersonal level, take good care of your relationships with others and treat others with respect. And at the organizational level, use to your advantage the frameworks in which you're working. And then let go of the rest. Let go of the mistakes of the past and the worries of the future. Don't spend too much time in the past or in the future. Look at what you can do *today*, here and now. The fuel that drives human performance is hope, and hope is something that can only grow in soil that is not poisoned by worry. Everybody needs a positive outlook on the future. So do what you can today, and rest assured you'll be okay.

Final Thoughts

Dear friend,

Thank you for reading *No Room for Shaky Hands*.

Please let me share some final thoughts with you. I hope the book was like going to an art museum and seeing a familiar painting with fresh eyes. What you saw may have been surprising, but after all there is only one thing that matters: did my humble book help you to provide better care to your valued patients?

The strategies described in this book have been effective for me, and I am sure they can work for you also. Life is too short to think about the stuff that doesn't work. I invite you to pick out the topics that will work for you and use them in your everyday practice.

Everybody has ideas to share. I'd love to hear your story. If you have interesting insights to tell about human performance in the operating room, please email me at noroomforshakyhands@gmail.com.

Also, I have a small favor to ask. It goes without saying that every first-time author faces the problem of creating credibility. Every author has to start with a small support group – a limited number of people who believe in the ideas, the writing, and the author.

Nowadays, the most important tools to get the momentum of a book going are online reviews. So, if you feel strongly about the value of this book, I would be eternally grateful if you posted a review on Amazon.

www.ingramcontent.com/pod-product-compliance
Lightning Source LLC
Chambersburg PA
CBHW051531170526
45165CB00002B/693